The Dynamics of British Health Policy

The Dynamics of British Health Policy

Stephen Harrison
David J. Hunter
Christopher Pollitt

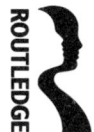

© Stephen Harrison, David J. Hunter, Christopher Pollitt, 1990
This book is copyright under the Berne Convention. No reproduction
without permission. All rights reserved.

First published in 1990

Reprinted in 1992 by Routledge
11 New Fetter Lane, London EC4P 4EE

British Library Cataloguing in Publication Data

Harrison, Stephen, 1947–
 The dynamics of British health policy.
 1. Great Britain. Health services. Policies of government
 I. Title II. Hunter, David J. III. Pollitt, Christopher
 362.10941

ISBN 0-415-09870-X

Typeset in 10 on 11 pt Bembo by
Columns Design and Production Services Ltd, Reading
Printed and bound in Great Britain by
Biddles Ltd, Guildford and King's Lynn

Contents

List of figures and tables	ix
Acknowledgements	xi
Series editor's preface	xiii
Introduction	xvii
1 Studying health policy	1
2 Funding health services	32
3 The management 'problem'	60
4 The NHS workforce	93
5 Measurement and evaluation	118
6 The dynamics of health policy	153
Annexe: The formal organization of the NHS	164
List of abbreviations	177
References	178
Index	194

List of figures

1.1	Three aspects of incrementalism	page	12
4.1	Gross pay comparisons, 1972–87		100
4.2	The pattern of medical careers		106
5.1	Evaluation concepts		120
A.1	Outline organization structure of English NHS, circa 1988		168
A.2	Proposed major NHS funding flows, 1992–3		173

List of tables

1.1	A comparison between rational comprehensive and incrementalist models of decisionmaking	10
2.1	Expenditure on UK health care as a percentage of GDP, 1979–86	34
2.2	The increasing numbers of the elderly	35
2.3	Trends in Health Service purchasing power and margins for service development	38
2.4	Health Services expenditure in the UK: selected years	40
2.5	Health expenditure: international comparisons as a percentage of GDP, 1984	42
2.6	UK independent hospitals: ownership 1979 and 1986	52
4.1	Growth of the NHS workforce	94
4.2	Movements in salary scale maxima of selected NHS staff groups: 1965–85 Index	98
4.3	Ratios of career medical posts to junior hospital medical posts, 1974–86	108
5.1	Key developments in evaluation, 1980–9	128

Acknowledgements

The three of us have taken an equal share of the work of writing this book, and of course we are jointly and entirely responsible for the views expressed and for any errors that appear. Nevertheless, there are many others who have contributed to our task, and we are glad to acknowledge them here. Linda Clark typed the final manuscript, and Nadia Davidson, Mary Dicker, Sylvia Greenwood, Anne Hunt, Jacqui Murgatroyd, Tina Stapylton and Jane Welsh all contributed to the typing of our (many) early drafts. John Hunt translated our messy Figures into masterpieces of clarity. Patricia Day (University of Bath), Jackie Holloway (Open University), Angela Jones (North-West Thames Regional Health Authority), Rod Rhodes (University of York), Liz Shore (University of London) and Jill Yeates (University of Sussex) provided helpful comments on various sections of the text.

Andy Shaw originally prepared Figure 4.1 for a postgraduate tutorial at the Nuffield Institute, and we are grateful for his permission to reproduce it. The staff of the Nuffield Institute Library saved us many hours of chasing references, and Claire L'Enfant, our editor at Unwin Hyman, showed great forbearance in the face of the several postponements of the copy date which were necessary in order to allow us to revise our analysis in the light of *Working for Patients*. Our thanks are due to all the above, but also to Hazel Yeomans, Annie Dearman, Adrian Jackson, and Jill Harrison, without whose support the book would not have been completed.

Series editor's preface

The crisis of the Swedish government in February 1990 over its proposals for drastic austerity measures, including the abandonment of its liberal sick leave policy, confirmed the scale of the malaise afflicting the post-war welfare state in Western Europe at the beginning of the 1990s. The last bastion of traditional social democratic welfarism, and the model for reformers from Dublin to Moscow, had fallen to the combined pressures of economic recession and political reaction. Pressures to curtail state expenditure on welfare first became apparent in the most stagnant economies of Europe – Britain, Belgium, France – in the mid-seventies. By the early nineties, even the prosperous countries of Scandinavia were putting the squeeze on welfare services. Throughout the West the ascendant ideology of the enterprise culture shattered the complacent consensus that had sustained four decades of expanding state welfare provision.

In Britain, all sides were dissatisfied with the old system of welfare. One of the earliest themes of what became known as Thatcherism was hostility to the 'dependency culture'. The ideologues of the new right denounced the 'nanny state' for its inefficient bureaucracy and profligate expenditure. On the other hand, many radicals and feminists were also critical of the remote welfare bureaucracies and their lack of accountability to users, workers and community pressures. However, it was the forces of Thatcherism that gained the initiative through three decisive election victories between 1979 and 1987. By the late eighties the government was confident that it had a mandate to impose its radical agenda on the public welfare system in Britain.

In the course of the eighties, the Conservative Government under Mrs Thatcher proceeded cautiously, carefully preparing public opinion for each anti-welfare step. However, every success gave ministers greater confidence for bolder measures and the process of unleashing market forces in public services steadily gathered momentum. The great sell-off of council housing was an early success which skilfully exploited the unpopularity of Labour local authorities and brought in substantial revenue. Cuts in social security and the general shift towards means-tested benefits were backed by media campaigns against 'scroungers'. In every sector of education resources were cut back and cost cutting measures introduced. A series of central government measures against local authorities resulted in a drastic deterioration in the quality of personal social services.

By the close of the decade the results of retrenchment and privatization were starkly evident. Homelessness and poverty among young people became a national scandal. The demoralization of staff in education was evident in a series of disputes at every level from nurseries to universities. A similar state of dissatisfaction was apparent in all areas of local government provision and throughout the voluntary sector. The revival of charity to compensate for the decline of public provision was a striking feature of welfare entering the 1990s.

The health service, the sphere of welfare enjoying the highest popular esteem despite its cost to the exchequer, proved the most resistant to the Thatcherite offensive. Conceding to the entrenched power of the medical profession as well as to the pressures of public opinion, Mrs Thatcher herself was obliged to proclaim that 'the NHS is safe with us' at the 1982 Conservative Party conference. However the 1989 White Papers *Working for Patients* and *Care in the Community*, introduced as a combined parliamentary bill at the beginning of 1990, served notice that the health service would no longer escape the chill winds of the capitalist market place.

In the fourth book in the **State of Welfare** series, Stephen Harrison, David Hunter and Christopher Pollitt note that before 1981 the government made little headway against the NHS. Indeed they observe that 'it was not even fighting'. In the mid-eighties, however, pressures on funding intensified, leading to a decline in expenditure in real terms at a time when the demands of an ageing population were growing rapidly. In the same period pressures to introduce the managerial principles of the retail sector – through the agency of top executives from Marks and Spencer (Rayner) and Sainsburys (Griffiths) – led to a series of inquiries, reports and measures to evaluate performance and raise efficiency. However, as the authors note, the radical edge of the new managerialism was blunted when it came up against the power of the medical profession to thwart government initiatives in the health service.

In response to the government's recognition that changes in the health service had turned out to be more a matter of form than substance, the 1989 white paper set out to tackle medical power head on. Its key proposal was the plan to create 'internal markets' within the health service, through 'self-governing' hospitals, 'budget-holding' general practices and a wider role for the private sector. The central aim of this drastic transformation in the structure of health service management and funding is to make doctors take responsibility for the financial consequences of their clinical decisions.

Can market forces provide a higher standard of health care? It is worth recalling the fact that the NHS was only introduced after the Second World War exposed the inadequacy of the market to provide modern health care, either in hospital or in the community, for the vast majority of the population. The evidence of the USA suggests that, not only does a more privatized system result in much greater inequality in standards of care, it also multiplies administrative costs and results in a much less cost-effective system. How such a system will work in Britain remains to be seen. As Harrison, Hunter and Pollitt indicate, the British government has in the past always pulled its punches when it comes to pushing through radical reforms against a resistant medical profession and established health care bureaucracy. Whether this will also be the fate of the current legislation remains very much an open question.

Mary Langan
The Open University

Introduction

It seems a long time since the three of us first mooted this book. Among other notable events, we have witnessed a general election, a major financial 'crisis' throughout much of the NHS, Sir Roy Griffiths' report on community care and, most recently, the White Paper *Working for Patients*, which resulted from the year-long prime-ministerial review of health services. The proposals contained in this last document seem likely to increase, rather than reduce, the diversity and complexity of the service that Aneurin Bevan put together in 1946, with which previous reorganizations had already sought to grapple. The same is true of the subsequent White Paper on community care, *Caring for People*.

Taken together, these and other changes have simultaneously reactivated public interest in health policy, yet accelerated the obsolescence of most of the existing texts which deal with the topic. The apparently high rate of change over the two years or so during which we have been writing has also had the benefit of providing us with a kind of running check on what we are saying. Though unlooked for, this has been a useful discipline which has obliged us to think very hard about the extent to which generalizations based on the experiences of the 1960s, 1970s and 1980s retain their validity in the 1990s.

The main aim of our book is to identify and analyse the dynamics of British health policy in the last two decades. As this cannot be achieved without the (explicit or implicit) use of theory, we have employed the first chapter in making our theoretical framework explicit. Our task also requires the use of descriptive materials; since there is an infinity of such material we have been obliged to make a selection, and Chapters 2 to 4 each deal with a policy area where there are persistent and crucial issues: funding, resource allocation, the balance between different types of service, the distribution of benefits across various categories of staff, and the evaluation and assessment of health care services, both during and after delivery. In a concluding chapter we attempt to draw the threads together and revisit the major theoretical questions raised at the beginning.

As has often been remarked, there can be few public services more basic to the quality of life in the civilized society than its health services. Precisely because of that pervasive importance, it continues to be quite impossible for health care in Britain to stand somehow 'above' or 'beyond' politics. Should additional proof of this be required one need only cast a cursory glance at other Western democratic societies in order to confirm that, in every single one, health is a prominent and perennially lively public issue. Once this inevitability is accepted the case for systematic study of what kind of political process is shaping health services becomes very strong. We hope, in what follows, to have made a contribution to that understanding. At a time when the social and political landscape is subject to such rapid change, the need for careful analysis and reflection has never been greater.

Steve Harrison
David J. Hunter
   University of Leeds, Nuffield Institute for Health Services Studies
Christopher Pollitt
   Open University, Faculty of Social Sciences

April 1990

1 Studying health policy

The aims of the book

The dominant concern of this book is to identify and analyse the main forces shaping United Kingdom health policies in the period since the early 1970s. It therefore provides neither a full history nor a comprehensive description of the institutions and procedures through which the health policy process flows. Rather, it concentrates on power relationships and the structures which facilitate and constrain them. Power relationships arise when one group or institution is dependent upon another. The nature of the dependency can vary widely – it may arise because one policy actor has control over money, or expertise, or commands the loyalty and trust of staff. Or it may be that a particular institution is endowed with formal (legal or administrative) authority to pronounce on specified issues. Such dependencies form intricate and cross-cutting patterns of power relationships – *interdependencies*, where the various parties can each constrain (or facilitate) the others' possibilities for action. For example, it is for the Cabinet, not the British Medical Association (BMA), to fix annually the total amount of money to be spent on the National Health Service (NHS). On the other hand, your general practitioner (GP), not your MP or your councillor, has the formal authority to prescribe (or not) drugs to treat any medical condition you bring to his or her attention. If GPs abuse that authority (by prescribing inappropriate drugs, for example) it is not the government, but the General Medical Council (GMC) which possesses the formal power to withdraw their licence to practise medicine. Thus it takes but little thought to see that 'policy' cannot be simply a matter of someone ('government'?) issuing orders which are then dutifully carried out. For example, studies of the effectiveness of Department of Health and Social Security (DHSS) circulars indicate that they were of very uncertain impact on the actual activities of the health authorities which received them (Ham, 1981). The NHS was founded on a complicated bargain between several parties (most notably the government, which brought to bear both money and powers of legislation, and doctors, with resources of monopoly, expertise, and popular esteem). In our study of the dynamics of health policy in the 1970s and 1980s we shall find a similarly complex web of mutual dependencies supporting a shifting assembly of pacts and bargains, both formally negotiated and tacitly understood.

It would be wrong, however, to imply that the parties to this bargaining process can strike any deal they please. 'Policy' is not so introverted or autonomous. For there are also structural constraints which limit the room for manoeuvre enjoyed by the various parties. The tightness or looseness of these constraints is a question occasioning much academic and political debate, but constraints there certainly are. Neither the government nor the BMA 'decided' to change the demographic structure in the direction of a much higher proportion of elderly persons. Nevertheless – in the United Kingdom as in other Western societies – once this shift began it had major implications for health services. Nor could the faltering rates of economic growth from the mid 1970s onwards fail to impact, sooner or later, on health care financing. Nor can any policymaker avoid the legacy of the past. An ageing hospital stock, a shortage of nurses or physiotherapists, a widespread problem of substance abuse – none of these contingencies can be dealt with in much under five years, even assuming the most radical measures and everything else 'standing still'.

We also wish to emphasize that we do mean UK health policies, and not merely English health policies. Some texts dealing with the NHS fail to acknowledge the extent to which there is not one, singular National Health Service, but several. England, Scotland, Wales and Northern Ireland differ markedly in terms of their respective organizational structures, resource inputs per capita and, indeed, in the health experiences of their populations (Hunter, 1982). In 1985/86 for example, Scotland received 19 per cent more NHS revenue finance per capita than England. Northern Ireland enjoyed 26 per cent more (Maynard, 1986, p.331). Despite this, compared with England, Scotland suffered significantly higher age-standardized mortality rates for both men and women. The relevant figures for 1979–80 and 1982–3 combined were (per 1,000 population), 5.43 (men, 20–64, England and Wales), 6.92 (men 20–64, Scotland); 2.17 (married women, 20–59, England and Wales), 2.89 (married women, 20–59, Scotland) (Whitehead, 1987, p.25). Organizational differences are equally marked. England, from 1974, sported a regional tier of health authorities interposed between the lowest tier and central government. The Scots, somehow, were able to do without this middle to the organizational sandwich (which they *lost* in 1974).

In England, Scotland and Wales throughout the 1970s and 1980s, criticism was heard of the baroque difficulties of successful coordination between health authorities and the social service departments of local authorities; in Northern Ireland, however, the two were combined in a single authority. There are many other examples – the intra-UK differences are of underexploited analytical potential. Finally there are also marked *policy* differences between the different countries – for example in the field of community care, the priority accorded to which for a long time seemed more substantial in England and Wales than in Scotland (Hunter and Wistow, 1987).

Understanding and explaining

What is involved in explaining how health policies are shaped and implemented? It is not possible to construct a single, 'correct', entirely 'objective' and value-free explanation of how health policies are concocted and carried out. Politicians and officials may sometimes claim that they can do this, but they are mistaken. The reason for discounting such claims will be given in a moment, but first it should be stressed that the impossibility of such an account does *not* mean that any explanation is as good as any other, or even that all explanations must be 'biased'.

One reason why value-free explanations are impossible is that choices of topic (what is to be explained) and of theory (how the explanation is to be constructed) are inevitably influenced by the investigator's values (for a standard exposition of these issues, see Bernstein, 1976). To decide that the large number of immigrant doctors in some medical specialties is a 'problem' or an 'issue worth investigating' is a value-influenced decision. Our values help determine what we see as 'problems' (Dunleavy and O'Leary, 1987, pp.334–43). Values also influence our choice of theory and approach. Some – especially politicians and officials – will stoutly deny any contact with 'theory' at all. In Britain this seems an especially popular conceit. The accusation that somebody is being 'theoretical' is frequently enough to gain the upper hand in debate. 'Let's stick to the facts', or 'in my experience' are gambits offered instead of the suspect procedure of 'theorizing'.

Unfortunately (for its *aficionados*) this blunt pragmatism, far from being a sturdy alternative to theorizing, usually turns out to be itself *implicit* theorizing, and often very poorly done at that. Every time some hard-bitten politician declares that progress can only come through negotiation and compromise; every time a civil servant says: 'You can make anything work so long as you send enough copies to enough people' (Pollitt, 1984a, p.152), they are expressing tacit theories – in these cases ones easily falsified by consulting the historical record. John Maynard Keynes, a man with wide experience in government and academe, observed that the most pragmatic people were, in their thinking, often 'slaves to some defunct economist' (Keynes, 1936).

There are at least two reasons why an apparently commonsense appeal to 'the facts' cannot escape, even if it can conceal, the process of theorizing. First, there is the awkward point that facts are only counted as facts according to some background rules. Thus a thoroughgoing behaviourist will not accept as 'evidence' an individual's descriptions of his or her emotional states and feelings because, the behaviourist's theory contains rules specifying that only observed behaviour, not reported mental states, can be regarded as reliable data. Similarly some Marxists will argue that the 'fact' that a majority of voters in a capitalist society have rejected the socialist candidates offered to them at the polls is not really a very meaningful or reliable 'fact' at all. It is simply the product of pervasive ideological conditioning which systematically conceals from voters the true nature of their interests, and offers instead the false but glittering promises of a 'free market society'. Thus, while factual evidence may certainly be used to cast doubt on the validity of a theory, theories also act back on the facts to some extent by defining in advance what will be accepted as reliable evidence and what will not.

Second, theories, whether implicit or explicit, privilege some facts over others. 'This is more important than that' they say. This is of great significance because the usual situation of the investigator seeking to explain some social phenomenon is one of gross factual overload. There is an infinity of facts that might be construed as relevant, and the investigator has to find some way of selecting out those which are most powerful in relation to the explanation sought. Why is Emma in such a bad mood at bedtime? Tired? Told off today at school by teacher? Food disagreed with her? Hasn't been hugged by her parents all week because they have been too busy and tired to think of it? These are all possibly relevant facts, but it takes a *theory* to establish which are likely to be the most important factors in Emma's life, and therefore which of the many bits of factual evidence is the one we should concentrate on. In this sense we are all tacit theorists all of the time. What is special about formal social science is that it includes an attempt to make the theorizing process particularly transparent and explicit. This is done so that it will be easier for others to see what we have done, to criticize our reasoning and (hopefully) to suggest more precise methods and/or more discriminating theories.

How, then, can one evaluate a theory and compare it with another? In the broadest terms there are three main tests. First there is the test of *comprehensiveness*, or scope. That is, how much does the theory purport to explain? Will it explain how all policies are made anywhere? Or only policymaking in the United Kingdom? Or only health policy in the United Kingdom? Or only health policy in the United Kingdom in times of economic growth, with a different method of policymaking appearing as soon as stagnation or decline sets in? Our own approach will seek to explain the health policy process in the United Kingdom since the early 1970s; it will therefore cover a period of acute economic crisis (roughly 1973–82) followed by one of slow, fragile and somewhat lopsided growth.

Second, there is the test of *coherence*. Is the theory internally logically consistent, or does it contain contradictions or ambiguities? Third, there is the test of the *consistency* of the theory with the evidence. Given that, as explained above, 'the evidence' is itself somewhat conditioned by the underlying theory, does it 'fit'? If not, is the inconsistency significant enough to throw doubt on the whole theoretical apparatus, and make some alternative theory more attractive? If a theory does not, or cannot, specify any empirical conditions under which it could be refuted, one must suspect that it is either circular, or a matter of faith, or both.

An 'explanation' – in our view – is thus a clearly articulated theory which is coherent, consistent with the evidence and of adequate scope to the questions being posed. In this book our own explanation focuses on power relationships. Policymaking does not conform to the requirements of 'rational planning' or 'comprehensive rationality' (Patten and Pollitt, 1980, pp.8–24). Instead 'policy' is better understood as the product of a bargaining process between a limited number of groups each one of which is interdependent (in a rich variety of ways) with the others. This bargaining 'network' or 'community' does change its membership somewhat from issue to issue and also – though only slowly – on given issues over time. But on the whole it has been a remarkably resilient and stable network, and this is why the implementation of radical (left or right) policies has been the exception rather than the rule. Seemingly major shifts in policy have been announced on several occasions, but subsequently the punches have been pulled.

The network, and its bargains, however, exist within a wider social and economic context. Even central government is often relatively impotent in the face of broad structural change. One of the key questions for this book, therefore, is whether changes already occurring in the policy environment seem likely fundamentally to upset relations 'inside' the health care community.

Even if punches have usually been pulled in the past, are we now on the brink of more punishing conflicts?

The existing literature

There is not enough space here for a thorough review of the health policy literature, but a brief selective commentary is essential if the reader is to understand 'where we are coming from'. In 1970 – roughly the beginning of the period under consideration – there were very few scholarly volumes dealing with the politics and policies of British health care. There were, of course, other kinds of literature – political biographies, histories of the medical profession, descriptive guides to the major institutions of health care and so on – but little with both an explicit policy focus and an academic/analytical intent. With hindsight this appears a remarkable absence, given the political significance, public popularity and fiscal 'weight' of the NHS. Since then, however, there has been a steady flow of texts (e.g. Allsop, 1984; Brown, 1975; Butler and Vaile, 1984; Ham, 1981 and 1985; Harrison, 1988a; Haywood and Alaszewski, 1980; Hunter, 1980; Klein, 1983; Lee and Mills, 1982). These differ considerably among themselves. For example some are more concerned with political dynamics, others with detailed institutional arrangements. Yet most of these works convey a broadly similar picture of how certain key relationships within the health sector seemed to work during the 1960s and 1970s. This we term the 'shared version', and it provides a useful starting point for our own account.

The 'shared version'

This common, or at least widely-shared account contained at least nine major features:
1 Health care politics are characterized as, in a broad sense, incrementalist. This means that changes in health service outputs (for example from an emphasis on acute hospital medicine to community-based forms of care) tend to be slow, and/or of narrow scope, rather than systematic or radical (Brown, 1979, p.205; Lee and Mills, 1982, p.179). This, in turn, derives from the distribution or power between the main 'actors' (ministers, civil servants, health authority members, NHS managers, doctors, other health care professionals and – occasionally – trade unions) and, institutionally, between 'centre' and 'periphery'.

2 The policy process is usually one of 'partisan mutual adjustment' (PMA), in which no one actor or institution can impose change, though several may be able to veto it (Ham 1985, ch. 4; Klein, 1983, pp.124–33; Lee and Mills, 1982, pp.118–20).
3 Within this PMA process, the medical profession continues to wield enormous influence at least in the 'defensive' sense of being able to frustrate those who wish to alter its training, conditions of service or patterns of practice (Allsop, 1984, p.226; Castle, 1980; Elcock and Haywood, 1980; Haywood and Hunter, 1982; Klein, 1983, pp.159–65; Long et al, 1987, Ch. 4).
4 The position of the lay health authority member is often weak relative to both clinicians and senior managers (Allsop, 1984, pp.229–30; Day and Klein, 1987, pp.76–104; Elcock, 1978, pp.392–6; Ham, 1985, p.158; Hunter, 1980, p.202; Ranadé, 1985, p.184).
5 The position of 'consumer' organizations is usually even weaker (Hallas, 1976, p.59; Lee and Mills, 1982, p.121). On the other hand their increased activity and 'density' over the last two decades signifies a broadening of the *dramatis personae* in the process of partisan mutual adjustment at least for certain *types* of issue (Allsop, 1984, pp.192–7; Ham, 1985, pp.108–10; Haywood and Hunter, 1982). However, these issues which are characterized by broader, pluralistic bargaining have tended not to be of the strategic type. Decisions concerning resource allocations, service priorities and the evaluation of effectiveness and efficiency remain fairly inaccessible to consumer groups.
   NHS management has tended to be highly 'introverted' (Harrison, 1988a, ch. 3).
6 The 'centre' (i.e. the 'health departments': see Annexe) possesses little direct operational control over the implementation of most national policies (Haywood and Alaszewski, 1980). It does, however, exercise considerable influence principally through (a) its control over the global sum of resources going into the NHS; (b) the allocation of this total between health authorities; (c) specific approval of large capital schemes and (d) the increasing practice (in England and Wales but less so in Scotland) of 'earmarking' revenue funds for particular purposes (Butler and Vaile, 1984, pp.77–88; Ham, 1985, pp.144–5; Pollitt, 1984b).
7 The role of health authority managers within this system of partisan mutual adjustment has usually been reactive. The emphasis has been on 'fire-fighting', diplomacy, conflict-avoidance and consensus-seeking, including maintenance of

some notion of 'fair shares' in allocative disputes (Ham, 1985, p.158; Harrison, 1988a, ch. 3; Hunter, 1980, pp.194–5; Schulz and Harrison, 1983; Stewart *et al*, 1980).
8 The policy inertia resulting from the distribution of power between the health departments, health authorities and the medical profession is further exacerbated by the extreme occupational complexity of the health service as a whole (Barnard and Harrison, 1986; Klein, 1983).
9 The whole complex and slow-moving edifice has been underpinned by an extremely durable political consensus (Allsop, 1984, p.37; Klein, 1983, pp.58, 146). This consensus has existed both internally and externally. It has existed internally in the sense that no subsequent government has directly challenged the basic deal struck between the then Labour government and the medical profession during the 'founding' period of 1946–8 (see Klein, 1983, ch. 1). Nor have either government or NHS managers tried to mount any major, frontal criticism of the 'medical model' of ill-health (Allsop, 1984, pp.203–12). It has existed externally in the high and continuing public popularity of the NHS, a popularity which has ensured it very high ratings (topped only – occasionally – by the monarchy) in numerous attitudes surveys concerning public institutions and services (Taylor-Gooby, 1985, pp.72–91).

This 'shared version' is to a large extent informed, sometimes explicitly, sometimes only implicitly, by what is known as incrementalism. It is important to understand at the outset that the incrementalist model is a general political science model which has proven useful in many different substantive policy sectors. Like most of the other models and theories of power relationships which will be discussed within these covers, incrementalism claims this wider applicability; one may find it in analyses of agricultural policy or education policy just as frequently as in studies of health policy.

Incrementalist theory, then, is very widely used. It is almost as widely misunderstood or misrepresented. A brief examination and critique should help clarify how far it can help us to understand British health policy, and where its usefulness stops.

In its origins (Lindblom, 1959) incrementalism is more a theory of the decisionmaking process than it is of outputs or impacts. Lindblom wanted to advance a model which he felt was a better description of most real-world decision processes than the much-advocated 'rational-comprehensive' model (Patten and Pollitt, 1980, pp.8–24). This rival model is of particular interest to us since many of its elements are echoed in efforts to 'reform' the NHS. Thus for example the stream of initiatives and changes flowing from the 1983 Griffiths Report (NHS Management Inquiry, 1983) to the 1989 White Paper (Department of Health *et al*, 1989b) frequently emphasized the need to clarify objectives, cost alternative means and monitor performance. The contrast between the two is summarized in Table 1.1.

Lindblom's 1959 article sparked off a long and intricate academic debate which became such a 'standard' element in policy analysis curricula that twenty years later he was persuaded to write a further piece, reflecting on where the argument had got to.

In that later article (Lindblom, 1979) he distinguished much more clearly between three different aspects of incrementalism. First, he wrote, there was incremental *politics* – the process of changing outcomes by small steps. Second, there was incremental *analysis* – a process of analysing policy problems which eschews grandiose attempts at synoptic ('big picture'/all the options) analysis and instead tackles problems one at a time and examines mainly options which are only incrementally different from the status quo. Finally, Lindblom separates *partisan mutual adjustment* from both incremental politics and incremental analysis. He defines PMA as fragmented or greatly decentralized political decision-making where policies are the resultants of attempts at mutual persuasion by the interests concerned, and outcomes (whether incremental or not) 'happen' rather than being the decision of some single or unitary authority. PMA is therefore 'to some extent a substitution of politics for analysis' (Lindblom, 1979, p.524) and does not *necessarily* occur alongside either incremental analysis or incremental politics.

The 'shared version': a critique

Clearly, Table 1.1 (adapted from the original 1959 article) refers to incremental *analysis*. One aspect of the 'shared version' that we accept is that incremental analysis *does* frequently seem to be a useful description of the health policy process as conducted by NHS managers and health authority (HA) members (Harrison, 1988a, ch. 3). But incremental analysis is a much less satisfactory model of government policy decisions. There it can be argued that, since as long ago as the early 1960s, the analysis of policy options has shown signs of becoming less and less 'incremental'. The accuracy, or usefulness of the notion of incremental *politics* is rather more difficult to assess. Again, it seems to 'fit' some levels and issues better than others. But there are also problems about

Table 1.1 *A comparison between rational comprehensive and incrementalist models of decisionmaking*

Rational Comprehensive Model	Incrementalist Model
1. Clarification of values and objectives distinct from and usually a prerequisite to empirical analysis of alternative policies	1. Selection of value goals seldom clearly defined. Usually closely, iteratively, intertwined with empirical analysis
2. Policy formulation approached through means–ends analysis, the ends already having been specified at step 1 (above)	2. Means and ends frequently not distinct, so means–ends analysis is often inappropriate or of limited scope
3. The best test of a 'good' policy is that it is, or can be shown to be, the most appropriate means to the desired and specified ends	3. A 'good policy' is one that commands wide agreement – or at least an absence of outright antagonism – among the interested parties. The same policy thus may sometimes commend itself to individuals or groups who actually seek different underlying objectives
4. Analysis is comprehensive – there is a systematic attempt to take every relevant factor into account	4. Analysis is limited in scope (few alternatives examined) and depth (underlying values are left ill defined). Agreement ('partisan mutual adjustment') is more important than analysis
5. 'Theory' is often prominent and heavily relied upon	5. A succession of limited comparisons (year-on-year within a given service, unit or specialism) reduces or eliminates reliance on 'theory'
6. Feedback is planned, systematic and promptly attended to	6. Feedback is seldom planned or systematic, and (partly because of the absence of clear objectives) it often fails to trigger changes in policy

Source: Adapted from Lindblom, 1959.

the concept of incremental change itself. To put it simply, how can the observer tell when an incremental change in outputs becomes a non-incremental change? Unless this dividing line can be drawn with a reasonable degree of precision the proposition 'this is incremental change' becomes virtually unfalsifiable. Lindblom does not entirely succeed in extricating himself from this difficulty when he points out that 'incrementalism varies by degrees' (Lindblom, 1979, p.517). The definition therefore remains somewhat subjective, and one person's increment may be another's radical change. Accepting this imprecision however, it is our view that incremental politics is not a bad description of the outcome of most health policymaking. Our evidence in favour of this interpretation will be set out in the descriptive chapters which follow. Note, however, that incremental politics does not necessarily mean conservative or slow-moving politics. As Lindblom himself argued: 'A fast-moving sequence of small changes can more speedily accomplish a drastic alteration of the status quo than can an only infrequent major policy change' (Lindblom, 1979, p.520). Such a sequence may, when adroitly handled, avoid major showdowns or trials of political strength (because no individual change is big enough to stir massive resistance) and can represent a kind of flexible, trial-and-error exploration of how far and fast it is possible to go. There is, however, one significant qualification to the usefulness of the incremental politics model, and that is that it seems to fit some *issues* much better than others. Thus while it may fit (say) inter-regional resource allocation since the mid-1970s fairly well, it does *not* adequately capture (say) policy change in relation to doctors' contracts of employment. We shall argue that the poor applicability of the incremental politics model to certain issues is connected with larger features of the power relations in health care, features which are best explained by the macro-level theories we shall introduce in the next section.

Finally, there is the role of partisan mutual adjustment; although we find plenty of incremental analysis in NHS policymaking, we do *not* find PMA a particularly useful conceptual tool. It does not, for example, describe the crucial relationship between doctors and managers very well (Harrison, 1988a). PMA suggests a rough equality or balance of influence and concession between major actors, but this is not the structure of bargaining we will show has obtained for a number of key health policy issues.

The relationships between the three aspects of incrementalism do not seem to have been very carefully explored. It is somewhat unfair of us to criticize the *coherence* of the 'shared version', since it is in a sense, our creation from the work of a number of authors (including ourselves). Nevertheless, incremental analysis, incremental politics and PMA are often apparently bundled together. Lindblom, on the other hand, asserts that there is no necessary connection, and we incline to this view, though with qualifications. It seems likely that in practice, PMA would lead to incremental politics; 'mutual adjustment' suggests small changes. It is also possible that PMA would encourage incremental analysis; if policymakers knew that powerful vested interests were certain to resist change, there would be little motivation for synoptic analysis. Incremental analysis need not, however, bear any relationship to incremental politics; synoptic analysis if it occurred, would in practice be highly likely to produce a series of small changes, even if these were aimed at some larger change in the long term. These connections are summarized in Figure 1.1.

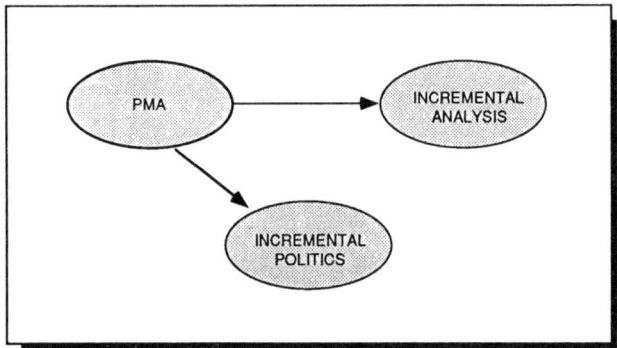

Figure 1.1 Three aspects of incrementalism.

The importance of these observations is considerable; they tend to reduce incremental analysis and incremental politics to the level of *description*, not explanation; it would be PMA (which it will be recalled, we do not consider to be consistent with research findings concerning NHS policy) that would constitute the explanation. In the absence of PMA, we have to find another explanation for incremental politics.

Two more general issues remain to be mentioned. First, even where incremental analysis, incremental politics or PMA will capture what actually happens, incrementalism concentrates too much on the *foreground* of the actual decision process and says too little about the background *environment* which frames the action, that is, it is not very *comprehensive*. Policy actors may mutually adjust but, as suggested earlier, they come into the arena far from equal. The consultants are usually more influential than the managers and the managers, in turn, seem to have greater influence than health authority members.

Explanation of these systematic inequalities requires us to go beyond the incrementalist 'frame', to a deeper level of analysis and theory, where the roots of power and influence may be directly addressed. In other words, the scope of the policy process extends well beyond the kind of local decisionmaking (especially that concerning resource allocation *within* health authorities) which provided the focus for much of the empirical research on which the 'shared version' was based. At national level, policy change may consist of steps rather than gradual creep, and the government has long possessed greater initiatory authority *vis-à-vis* the representative bodies of the medical profession than most local managers have enjoyed with their local consultant body. National level policy dynamics do not necessarily mirror local patterns and, notoriously in the case of the NHS, the local medical élite does not always fall in line with agreements reached by the BMA or the Royal Colleges at national level.

A second limitation of the incrementalist model, closely connected with the first, is that it does not take us very far in understanding why some issues arrive on decision agendas and others never reach them. Again, we need to go to a deeper level of analysis, to examine the distribution of power and influence. In this case it is the second face of power we are interested in. The first face concerns the power to win the arguments concerning issues on the agenda and to get things done. The second face concerns the more subtle business of preventing some issues from reaching the formal agenda in the first place (Bachrach and Baratz, 1970; Lukes, 1977). Thus for example, treating GPs as salaried NHS employees rather than independent contractors was effectively off the agenda for a long time after the original political compromises that constituted the NHS. Or again, when the 1975–6 Resource Allocation Working Party (RAWP) was working out its resource allocation formula, primary care was quickly excluded from its scope because it promised to be such a 'hot potato' (to quote one member of the Working Party) that it threatened to delay and ensnare the whole process.

Beyond the 'shared version': theories of the distribution of power

The ideas of the first and second faces of power come from the political theory literature. This is a highly relevant body of writing for an exploration of the environment within which the foreground processes of NHS decisionmaking take place. On the whole, however, most health policy specialists have *not* made much use of this potential. Doctors and health service specialists tend not to be very familiar with political theory while political scientists have often been concerned with more obviously conflictual topics such as party political competition or macroeconomic policy.

Recently, however, a few authors have begun to bridge this divide. Allsop (1984), for example, gives brief consideration to four critiques of the health care arena – professional dominance, political economy, Marxism and the radical right. Ham (1985) concludes his text with a similarly brief account of three theoretical approaches to the distribution of power; Marxist, pluralist and structuralist. He concludes that each has some merit but none is adequate by itself. His recommendation is for more work on linking these theories to each other, and on connecting macro theory to specific policy issues. We endorse this view, and an exploration of the distinctive insights afforded by such theories is a prominent feature of the present text.

This leads us to the problems of theory choice. Here we are severely constrained. It is impossible to summarize all the major political theories in the available space. Even if one selects (as we shall do in a moment) a limited sub-set of those theories there is still only room for a potted summary of some of their more salient aspects. Readers who wish to pursue these theoretical aspects more deeply are therefore strongly advised to look beyond the present text – we would particularly recommend Dunleavy and O'Leary (1987) and Held (1987, Part 2).

The theoretical approaches that we have chosen to introduce are as follows:

- Neo-pluralism
- Public choice (which includes what Allsop refers to as the 'radical right critique')
- Neo-élitism (which includes both 'liberal corporatism' and what Allsop terms the 'professional dominance critique')
- Neo-Marxism

Neo-pluralism
Classic pluralists see power as being fairly widely distributed in society, and as stemming from possession of a variety of resources (money, expertise, authority, votes and so on). But to make these resources 'count' it is necessary to organize, manoeuvre and bargain for one's interests. Pressure groups and lobbying activity

still remain a central focus for neo-pluralists, and the state is seen as having a special role in 'refereeing' this constant process of interest group bargaining, coalition-forming and coalition-splitting. However, unlike classic pluralists, neo-pluralists do not see this process as necessarily being more or less equally open to all interests who trouble to organize themselves. Nor do they see the state as, typically, a neutral or fairly passive, actor. On the contrary, the neo-pluralists, impressed by the growth of large corporations and large-scale interventionist bureaucratic government, see the policy-bargaining process as often rather lop-sided. Big business occupies an especially privileged position, not least because through its simultaneous – and highly organized – control of wealth, employment and expertise, it can often effectively veto public policies which it perceives as threatening (Lindblom, 1977; Dahl, 1985). But the state is also a force to be reckoned with. As it has grown and extended the scope and depth of its interventions in civil society, so it has acquired interests of its own, and an extended and powerful bureaucratic apparatus.

The old idea of politically controlled line bureaucracies has been displaced by complicated networks of decentralised, professionally-run agencies. When corporations deal with government, therefore, there is no clash of organisational forms, but instead a ready understanding and a high degree of congruence in administrative arrangements (Dunleavy and O'Leary, 1987).

Correspondingly, there has been a decline in the relative influence of representative political institutions such as Parliament and the political parties. Yet there is still a range of issues where democratic processes can predominate, and where new groups and interests may enter the arena and command some influence. These issues are of two main types. The first are those where the root interests of big business are not directly threatened. The second are major, 'history-making' issues, where massive media attention and public interest create a democratic counterweight to the processes of 'private' oligopolistic mutual accommodation and bargaining between experts and their bureaucratic employers.

Despite these more classically 'pluralist' exceptions, neo-pluralists concentrate their main attentions on the predominance of more closed, oligopolistic policymaking. Thus they have become very interested in the concept of 'policy networks', inhabited by government departments, professional bodies, major non-departmental public agencies, large corporations and so on (Rhodes, 1988; Wright, 1988). Here 'business as usual' means regular but largely private bargaining and compromise.

This model of 'how things are' appears to offer some immediate insights into health policymaking. On the surface the health care policy arena is characterized by a large community of competing groups. The British Medical Association says this, the Association of Community Health Councils says that, BUPA (the leading private medical insurance group) says something else, MPs have their say and even the Department of Health often displays more than one perspective. But within this diversity lurk tighter, more exclusive networks which exert a strong, continuing influence over a wide range of health policy issues. The members here are senior officials in the health departments, chairs and senior managers in the health authorities and the representative institutions of the medical professions (Haywood and Hunter, 1982). Thus it often seems that the deliberations of representative political bodies, including Parliament, are much less important in shaping the policy process than these endless jockeyings-for-position among the smaller community which inhabits the insider networks. It is through such networks, according to neo-pluralists, that political *integration* – or at least the avoidance of all-out conflict – is delivered.

Other, less obvious, features of the neo-pluralist model also seem to explain aspects of the policy dynamic. The special influence of big business may not at first seem obvious in a nationalized health service such as that in the United Kingdom. Yet, behind the scenes, there are many examples of how difficult it is for governments to regulate corporate power, even when in some sense they want to. The story of the painfully slow and incremental attempts by the DHSS and its predecessor department to control the prices of drugs supplied to the NHS by the major pharmaceutical companies is one such. The failure – despite being in the position of being a very large customer indeed – to achieve satisfactory cost control dragged on from the early 1950s well into the 1980s, punctuated by occasional inquiries, repeated renegotiations and the odd scandal. A second example is the equally tortuous tale of governments' attempts to discourage cigarette smoking. Despite its long-attested association with a variety of serious medical conditions (expensive ones from the NHS's point of view) the DHSS moved very cautiously indeed and bent over backwards to achieve voluntary agreements with the tobacco companies. More recently the government has clearly been reluctant to give vigorous publicity to scientific evidence concerning the health effects of a number of foodstuffs, at least partly because of pressure from agribusiness interests. Notice that these examples fall well outside the domain of the 'shared version'. As indicated above, one of the advantages of broader political power models such as those under consideration in this section is precisely that they direct attention to such issues, which may not be the stuff of headlines in the way that hospital closures or waiting lists or nurses' pickets are, but which nevertheless impact extensively on the health of the population and on the finance and operation of the NHS.

Finally, what appear to be the weaknesses of neo-pluralist theory? Here it is useful to reintroduce our three criteria of *scope, coherence* and *consistency*. In terms of scope neo-pluralism tends, in the hands of most of its exponents, to be limited to what one might call the foreground of political action. The focus is on manoeuvre, tactics, who said what to whom and when, and how this affected the outcomes of the 'game'. The resources of the various players are usually taken into account, but little or nothing may be said about the deep structures, i.e. demographic and technological change, the ideological climate or the background pattern of ownership and control. Because neo-pluralists do not concentrate on these constraining factors the impression may be given that decisionmaking processes are more indeterminate, unpredictable and open-ended than the actual history of outcomes might indicate. On the other hand neo-pluralism does at least represent an advance on classic pluralism in this respect, since it has begun to acknowledge and explore the roots of the especially influential part so often played by big business.

Against the coherence criterion neo-pluralism seems fairly robust. Well-crafted pluralist accounts do not contain any glaring internal incoherences, and would not have survived as such a strong tradition in political studies if they had. There is, however, an area of ambiguity concerning the operation of structural constraints of the kind referred to above. Pluralism does not seem to offer any convincing way of discriminating between actions that are necessary (inescapable) and those which are contingent, or chosen. Its vagueness on this point probably contributes to the tendency of pluralist accounts to imply relative open-endedness in decision processes.

Neo-pluralism scores well with respect to the consistency criterion, at least in the sense that it can produce accounts which read very 'realistically'. However, some critics find this unsatisfactory because it is hard to see how such accounts could be falsified, other than on grounds of crude factual error. There is a sense in which, because of the multi-causal, indeterminate character of the theory, pluralist accounts can degenerate into blow-by-blow story-telling from which it is very hard to extract any larger patterns of constraining and enabling forces. Each episode becomes almost unique, and personality factors can always be deployed to explain (or explain away) any unusual outcomes.

Public choice theory

Public choice theory has grown and thrived partly as a critique and rejection of both classical pluralism and neo-pluralism. Pluralism emphasizes the democratic possibilities of group processes, negotiation and compromise. Its usual approach is basically inductive, so it begins with direct observations of the 'realities' of everyday politics and policymaking and theorizes from these. Public choice theory, by contrast, is suspicious of the outcomes of group bargaining, lays great stress on the importance of *individual* choice, and often proceeds by way of deductive reasoning from a few simple hypotheses about how individuals will behave. At the heart of most public choice theory is the neo-classical economist's model of the utility-maximizing individual.

The public choice approach is usually (but not exclusively – see Dunleavy and O'Leary, 1987, p.75) associated with the values, policies and programmes of the new right (or radical right). Within this affiliation there are at least two divergent strands, the neo-liberals and the neo-conservatives. The latter, particularly prominent within the moral majority movement in the United States, are enthusiastic to restore what they see as traditional moral values. Thus they are in favour of the patriarchal family, organized Christianity, and patriotism and are virulently opposed to (for example) homosexual rights, abortion, and socialism in all its manifestations (Hoover and Plant, 1989). For our present purposes, however the neo-liberals are of greater interest. The neo-liberal analysis is fundamentally hostile to the welfare state, including the NHS. In this view the welfare state has become an unsustainable burden on the economy as a whole. Further, the organizational forms and processes of the welfare state have become a threat to the liberty and freedom of many individuals.

To understand this approach it is necessary to appreciate the accompanying analysis of the trends in the state–civil society relationship. One of the founding texts on this subject is Hayek's *The Road to Serfdom* (1986) originally published in 1943. Hayek was intensely suspicious of any attempts at centralized state planning or regulation. The proper function of the state was to formulate and implement a limited number of general laws on which there was widespread agreement. These might be laws concerned with safeguarding the rights of the individual, protecting private property and maintaining public order. Once the state stepped beyond this role and attempted detailed planning and regulation, particularly of the kind that was directed against specific groups in society rather than at the citizen body as a whole, then freedom was in danger. Neither could the state ever amass and organize the enormous quantities of detailed information that it would need if it were to be effective in such an expanded role. Unfortunately, however, many states had been tempted to do just this. Huge planning and regulating bureaucracies had sprung quickly into being and had soon begun to amass power to themselves, eroding the individual's freedom of action and choice and creating a culture of dependency. These bureaucracies developed their own momentum, since the further growth and expansion of their services was very much in the sectional interests of the groups that dominated them, i.e. the service providers themselves. What is more, the encroachment of bureaucratic planning onto social territory previously governed by market mechanisms led to serious decreases in efficiency.

During the late 1960s and 1970s Hayek's analysis was taken up and elaborated by a growing number of academics and politicians. For example, Niskanen produced an extended analysis of public sector bureaucracies which suggested that they had an almost universal tendency to oversupply their services (Niskanen, 1971). This was because senior officials, like everyone else, attempted to maximize their own utility and, this, in Niskanen's view, took the form of maximizing the size of their departmental budgets. The world economic crisis of the mid-1970s seemed to confirm the worst fears of the new right. Faltering economic growth was confidently attributed to the burden of overblown public welfare. In Britain, and to an even greater degree in the United States, it was open season for attacks on the parasitic, costly, self-interested bureaucracies of education, health care and the personal social services (Pollitt, 1990). The title of a booklet by a British new right theorist captures the thrust of this critique very well – *Breaking the Spell of the Welfare State* (Anderson et al, 1981). At about the same time another prominent new right author opined as follows:

> Not only double but multiple standards are the only way to raise standards for all – especially for the poorest. The search for an equal service NHS is vain as long as people differ, as long as they put their loved ones before abstract political dogmas, as long as incomes differ, and as long as incomes rise. The whole issue of equality has been confused with that of poverty, and both have obscured the overriding objective of liberty . . . Many in Britain would pay more, but the NHS stops them. Yet this is the great hope for the future; that more and more people will voluntarily spend more than the state now allows them to

do. And that will be the source of the additional funds for medicine. The method of the NHS is compulsion – taxation (Seldon, 1980, p.145).

Given this theory, which – it should be noted, takes an opposite view of the problem from Niskanen – the remedies are fairly obvious. First, the sphere of planning must be diminished and that of the market mechanism increased. Thus, private health care should be encouraged, while the provision of any additional services by public health care agencies should be severely restricted. The individual will be better served in a system where she or he can choose to go elsewhere (the power of exit) than in one that relies exclusively on pluralistic bargaining between organizational groups (the power of voice) (Hirschman, 1970). Various actions can therefore be taken to reduce the negative effects of the welfare state. First, public bureaucracies can be divided up into two or more units which can then be obliged to compete with one another, mimicking the competition of the market place. Second, wherever possible, public services can be required to charge for the benefits they offer, thus deterring frivolous use and 'free riders'. Third, the monopoly power of individual public service professions (very much including the medical profession) can be weakened by changing their terms and conditions of employment, by encouraging them to advertise and compete with one another, and by subjecting them to the quasi-market disciplines of performance indicators and other types of managerial monitoring and control.

During the 1980s these tactics have been applied to many public services, including health care, by both Thatcher and Reagan administrations (Pollitt, 1990). The internal market proposed for the NHS in the 1989 White Paper clearly had its origins in new right thought (Department of Health et al, 1989b). Yet neither the British nor the American government has yet been able to implement the full manifesto implied by the new right analysis (see for instance Hoover and Plant, 1989; Klein, 1985). Nevertheless, their policies have contained many echoes of new right thinking. Hospital catering, cleaning and laundry services have been put out to competitive tender. Private health care facilities have been encouraged and taxation rules for private health insurance eased. Health authorities have been urged to sell off buildings and land. The 1989 White Paper on the NHS gave official blessing to the concept of the efficiency-seeking self-governing hospital and to competition (both in primary and secondary care) for patients. Systems of performance indicators have been introduced to encourage comparisons between the

English DHAs and RHAs. A variety of schemes has been introduced for encouraging, or enforcing greater 'efficiency' and, simultaneously for paying greater attention to the sensibilities of the individual health care 'consumer'. These measures have not, in total, amounted to a rolling back of the NHS, but they are at least indicative of public choice theory aspirations, and, therefore, of a significant shift in ideological climate.

When public choice theory is subjected to the same tests as those we applied to neo-pluralism the contrast in its characteristics becomes very clear. The scope of public choice theory is at once rather broad yet extraordinarily narrow. It is broad in the sense that at least some public choice theorists believe their model can explain very general trends in both policymaking and economic development. As we have noted, the theory offers an account of the growth of the welfare state and of multifarious impacts which this growth is said to have had both on the economy and the attitudes and behaviour of different groups in society (such as welfare beneficiaries, public servants). Yet at the same time this account is mounted on a very narrow base, namely a few fairly simple postulates about how individuals are motivated and how their cognitive processes then determine which courses of action they will pursue. Thus there are many aspects of the policy process about which public choice theory has little or nothing to say. In the health care field, for example, what of altruism, professional ethics or the concept of public service? Public choice accounts are usually silent on these matters, or go to some lengths to try to reconceptualize them as subtle forms of self-interest maximization.

Public choice theory scores highly on coherence, partly because of this simple model at its core. It is a much more compact, clearly specified model than neo-pluralism, and will more readily yield falsifiable predictions about what is likely to happen in a given situation. This ingenious simplicity may partly account for the success it has had when popularized by politicians and pundits. On closer inspection, however, it appears that (at least) Niskanen's version of budget-maximizing bureaucrats contains some damaging imprecisions and inconsistencies (see, for instance Goodin, 1982). For example, even if bureaucrats *are* obsessed with their budgets, their motivations may vary considerably depending on whether it is the headquarters core budget, the bureau budget (core plus money paid directly to the private sector, such as contracts), the programme budget (bureau budget plus monies passed to other public sector bodies) or the super-programme budget (as above plus spending by other agencies which the bureau *controls*). Close examination of the logic of bureaucratic

conduct suggests that senior civil servants may not wish to maximize the programme budget at all, although they will be very concerned with both the core budget and the super-programme budget (Dunleavy, 1989).
The relationship between public choice theory and empirical evidence is, however, problematic. One price to be paid for elegant simplicity is evidently that there are many aspects of the real world which it explains badly or not at all: 'There is no place for people to work in their favourite war stories' (Goodin, 1982, p.24). What is more, the seduction of reasoning from first principles has kept many, perhaps most, public choice theorists from doing much applied empirical work to test their hypotheses. Where this has been done it is by no means clear that the findings bear out the predictions (Dunsire et al, 1988). In the United States, for example, the introduction of Medicare prospective payment systems, which should have strengthened hospital management and compelled doctors to practise in an economically more efficient manner, evidently failed to have anything like the expected impact (Weiner et al, 1987). Organizational and political processes proved more resistant to changed economic incentives than had been supposed.

Neo-élitism

According to this theory power is not distributed at all equally in our society. Rather it is disproportionately concentrated in the hands of a limited number of élites. These élites may be functional or occupational groups. They may compete among themselves, but are likely to join forces to resist any attempt extensively to broaden participation in decision making or make a reality of 'mass democracy'. Thus élite theory is focused on *group* behaviour rather than the model of individual behaviour which underlies public choice theory. The reasons why inequalities leading to the formation of élites arise may be very various (and there are differences of view among élite theorists about this), but once the inequalities are there, a virtually inevitable set of processes will enable a favoured group to further enhance its position in some particular field. For example, Michels, an early and influential élite theorist, formulated an 'iron law of oligarchy' (Michels, 1915). Roughly, this 'law' posited that large groups cannot take complex decisions so they are obliged to appoint leaders with some delegated authority. Once appointed, however, these leaders rapidly diverge from the rank and file in terms of their specialist information and skills. They are able to create increasing areas of discretion and, as their own power grows, it becomes increasingly important to them to hang onto that power, even if that may involve manipulating the rank and file.

While all élite theorists emphasize the importance of élites in the policy process, they by no means agree on how to value this state of affairs. Some think it inevitable, and, if they have proposals for reform, concentrate these on improving the quality of élite recruitment processes. Others believe the current degree of élite dominance is not necessary, and propose improved means of holding élites to public account.

One recent variety of élite theory which is of particular interest to students of health policy is *liberal corporatism* (Dunleavy and O'Leary, 1987 pp.193–7). In this model the state, in an attempt to ease its problems in managing an increasingly complex civil society, offers favours and status to a few selected interest groups in return for their agreement to behave in 'moderate' ways and to help in disciplining the rank and file. This arrangement is quite distinct from pluralism:

> *Pluralism* can be defined as a system of interest representation in which the constituent units are organized into an unspecified number of multiple, voluntary, competitive, nonhierarchically ordered and self-determined ... categories which are not specially licensed, recognised, subsidised, created or otherwise controlled by the state ... *corporatism* can be defined as a system of interest representation in which the constituent units are organized into a limited number of singular, compulsory, noncompetitive, hierarchically ordered categories, recognised or licensed (if not created by) the state and granted a deliberate representational monopoly ... in exchange for observing certain controls on their selection of leaders and articulating of demands and supports (Schmitter, 1974, pp.93–6, italics added).

Thus in this model both Parliament and political parties take side seats. The big deals worked out between the state and the 'peak associations' (the favoured, élite, organized groups) and then 'sold' to the rank and file and the general public. However, not all sectors of society are necessarily corporatized in this way, and in practice not every single one of Schmitter's criteria may be met even in those sectors where there is an élite interest group favoured by the state.

The relevance of all this for health policy is immediately clear. The medical profession is surely just a state-licensed élite – at least for the purposes of its national-level dealings with government. The state uses its legislative authority to prohibit non-members of the profession effectively from practising medicine, and the profession undertakes to control and discipline its members in a wide variety of ways. Various professional bodies such as the BMA and the Royal Colleges (of Physicians, Surgeons and so on) are in close and constant contact with ministers and government officials (see Castle, 1980 and Crossman, 1977). They are routinely consulted on matters going far beyond the terms and conditions of service of their members. No organization representing patients enjoys anything like this degree of influence. Other health professions also enjoy elaborate consultative arrangements and recognition as the sole official representatives of their functional interests, but do not play the intimate role in policymaking achieved by the medical profession itself.

An alternative explanation of the same phenomenon is provided by the notion of 'ideological corporatism' (Dunleavy, 1981). Instead of stressing the government bargain with interest groups which is the starting point of liberal corporatism, ideological corporatism stresses a shared view of the world, which makes it seem unnecessary for government to regulate the professions in any more than a general way:

> The effective integration of different organisations and institutions . . . by the acceptance or dominance of an effectively unified view of the world . . . [T]he active promotion of changes in ideas rests quite largely with individual professionals . . . bargained or negotiated compromises will be relatively rare (Dunleavy, 1981, pp.8–9) . . . the distinction between formulation and implementation may dissolve altogether . . . so that policy is just what professionals in the field do (Dunleavy, 1981, p.13; see also Lipsky, 1980).

Élite theory therefore directs attention towards the protected world of peak associations and the corresponding departments of government. It illuminates ways in which, though sometimes disagreeing vigorously over particular measures, these two sides usually sustain and support each other's authority. It suggests the possibility that policy changes need not always be incremental, because just a few of the myriad interest groups in the world of health care matter much more than the others so, if these few can be persuaded (or can themselves persuade the government), then more radical or sweeping changes may be achieved. But it also suggests that problems relating to the original 'bargain' between the government and the medical profession may be especially difficult to resolve. Thus, for example, élite theorists would not be surprised to find that reforms involving substantial dilution of the medical profession's 'clinical freedom', or their rights to practise privately even when holding NHS positions, have consistently remained in the 'non-starter' category. Some élite theorists, however, do entertain the possibility of serious competition between élites. One such piece of work is Alford's (1975) influential 'structural interest theory'.

In outline, structural interest theory posits that the field of health care can be conceptualized as consisting of a number of broad interests; while each of these may display some internal conflict, each is defined in terms of the extent to which its interests are 'served or not served by the way in which they fit into the basic logic and principles by which . . . institutions . . . operate' (Alford, 1975, p.14). Interests may be 'dominant', 'challenging', or 'repressed'. Dominant interests are those served by the existing system; their strategies are therefore basically defensive, and they may be supported by general societal approval of their status. Challenging interests are created and sustained by societal changes such as in technology and markets; their interests lie in changing the *status quo*. Repressed interests are the opposite of the dominant in that the nature of institutions systematically ensures that they are not served, though from time to time specific pressure groups may arise within the repressed interest, and may achieve isolated changes.

In Alford's own case studies of health care in New York City, doctors are seen as a 'professional monopoly', and hence as the dominant interest; the owners and managers of health care institutions, together with relevant government actors and insurers are seen as 'corporate rationalizers', challenging the dominant medical interest with attempts to introduce planning systems and cost controls. Finally, the 'community population' is the repressed interest: those people who cannot afford health insurance and yet do not qualify for government welfare benefits. A number of writers (see, for instance, Allsop, 1984; Ham, 1985) have argued for the relevance of this model to the NHS. The *scope* of élite theory is potentially quite broad (the sum total of relationships between élites and other élites, and between élites and the masses, across the whole of society) but in practice it is frequently rather narrow. The typical example of the *genre* is probably a study (such as Alford's) of one particular élite, and its relations with other actors in the same sector, including élites of state officials. A more general limitation is that élite theory is overwhelmingly a theory of political and organizational processes; it has nothing distinctive to say about economic and technological change, other than, perhaps, that whatever economic and technological changes occur, élites will do their best to suppress those which threaten them and take advantage of those which will enhance their power.

The coherence of élite theory is typically less well defined – or at least less obvious – than that of public choice theory. While the central process by which the gap between leaders and rank and file opens up may be clearly spelt out, the ultimate limits to élite power are left rather vague. That some élitism exists seems an almost trivial hypothesis, while the hypothesis that every sphere is élite-dominated is too crude. What, then, are the mechanisms which determine how much élitism will exist in a given set of circumstances, and of what type? There seems to be no single, simple response to this, no counterpart to the elegant model of the utility-maximizing individual which powers public choice theory. Élitism, here, is a broad church, more like pluralism, at least in the sense that many diverse factors may be seized upon to explain a particular case.

This diversity of explanation gives élite theory a flexibility which permits it to generate accounts of the real world which seem highly consistent with the facts. Indeed, élite explanations may have a special appeal for those of us who are predisposed to suspect a 'hidden hand' behind events. It is often tempting to believe that public affairs are principally driven by one or another form of insider dealing. By the same token, however, access is frequently a problem for élite theory researchers. If there are élites who are fixing things behind the scenes in their own interests, they are unlikely to welcome prying academics. For example, there is strong anecdotal evidence that, prior to the 1979 election, Mrs Thatcher's views on health were strongly influenced by certain consultants and that their advice, in turn, directly reflected their own experience and interests as clinicians in particular, high-prestige specialisms, with extensive private practices. It would be very difficult, however, to get beyond anecdote or 'unattributable briefing'; the individuals concerned are hardly going to volunteer the details of what was said and why.

A further point about the consistency of élite theory is of particular significance for this book. It is that distinctions between levels need to be carefully applied to élite studies. The medical profession, for example, may be an élite, but it is also an internally divided one in which the divisions seem to operate in different ways at different levels. Government/BMA/Royal Colleges deals may be struck at the national level, but the 'peak associations' may not be able to 'deliver' the rank and file. Some examples of this are analysed in Chapter 4. At local level, also, the dominant impression can sometimes be one of warring medical specialisms, each fighting for its territory and resources rather than a unified, disciplined entity.

Neo-Marxism and the 'new left'

Orthodox Marxism often took a rather mechanistic view of the state–civil society relationship. Civil society was characterized by a massive and continuing conflict between a dominant capital-owning class and a virtually propertyless working class which was obliged to sell its labour to the former class in order to survive. The terms on which the capitalists purchased this labour were exploitative, hence the unremitting class antagonisms. In this scheme of things the state was usually portrayed as the instrument of the capitalist class, either suppressing working-class resistance with coercion, buying it off with welfare concessions or defusing it with ideological seductions to national unity, patriotism or the common interest.

For neo-Marxists and others on the new left the picture is both more complex and more plastic. (In the interests of brevity we are having to lump together a number of shades of opinion here; it is no longer clear where Marxism ends and other forms of radical analysis begin.) Class antagonisms and massive inequalities of power remain the root characteristics of capitalist society, but the class structure itself is conceived in more fractured and variegated terms. Élites may, as in the neo-élitist model, be prominent. But whereas in that model élites may arise through economic, technological, social or other processes, in neo-Marxism élites are almost always related to the underlying class structure. The role of the state is also seen very differently. Instead of being the simple tool of rather monolithic capitalist interests, the state becomes a battleground over which various class interests struggle (Poulantzas, 1978). Even if constrained in the last resort by the need to promote the accumulation of capital, for most purposes the state has developed a degree of relative autonomy from any one class interest. Exactly how much autonomy (what defines the last resort) has been a matter for agonized debate, but the vulgar Marxist image of the state as just the bankers' cat'spaw has conclusively disappeared from academic Marxism. Perhaps not surprisingly, the new left has had to modify its theories in order better to come to terms with some of the same prominent features of modern societies that have concerned the new right. The left, too, sees the liberal democratic state as unable to cope with the plurality of demands made of it (Offe, 1985, p.314). It acknowledges the significance of the global economic changes of the mid-1970s, even if it attributes these changes to a different set of causes. It also acknowledges that centralized state bureaucracies can easily become rigid, unwieldy, and to a degree self-serving. 'Client' encounters with these services may often be bewildering, stigmatizing or downright unpleasant. Fabian-style national, professionalized service delivery organizations are no longer seen as the automatic response to a wide range of social problems. Indeed, 'The state is inescapably locked into the maintenance and reproduction of the inequalities of everyday life and, accordingly, the whole basis of its claim to distinct allegiance is in doubt' (Held, 1987, p.256).

This, of course, is where the new left begins to sound very different from the new right. For the left the state, far from threatening the vigour of capitalism, is ultimately its captive. For example, if the state tries radically to increase welfare spending it has to raise taxes. This impacts upon the business community which then 'loses confidence', fails to invest, and thereby provokes an economic crisis. The likely electoral consequences of the economic crisis oblige the government of the day to scale down its welfare plans. Or again, the new left argues that it is no accident that occupational health and safety was for long (and – some assert – still remains) a relatively neglected area, outside the NHS. For of all aspects of health care this is the one where the requirements of good health most obviously and immediately collide with the capitalist drive to minimize costs and maximize profits.

While neo-Marxists therefore still see the capitalist class as exercising strong constraints on the state's ability to expand public expenditure, they have begun to make significant distinctions between different categories of such expenditure. Three basic categories are identified, distinguished by their larger social functions. First there is the social expenses category. This comprises state expenditure aimed at the basic function of maintaining order, for example by providing a police force. Second, social investment expenditure supports the process of capital accumulation, and is therefore regarded relatively favourably by those fractions of capital which are likely to derive direct benefit from it. An example here would be the provision, by the state, of an efficient transport system, or energy supply system, closely geared to the needs of business and industry. The third category is social consumption expenditure and includes health and welfare expenditure. The function of this type of expenditure is to maintain the workforce in at least minimal functional order and, most importantly, to 'legitimate' the entire capitalist system by making it appear that the state cares and is genuinely trying to promote a fair and just society for all. Although this kind of classification has been strongly criticized (Dunleavy and O'Leary, 1987, pp.251–3) it is of some interest in raising the important point that, whether the NHS is actually terribly effective or efficient or not, its very *existence* has provided governments with a powerful legitimating symbol. Even Mrs Thatcher, for whom the philosophical foundations of the NHS would appear to be considerably at odds with her own ideology, felt it prudent, before the 1983 general election campaign, to claim that the NHS was 'safe in our hands'. Governments may thus face conflicting pressures over welfare state funding at a time of economic crisis (O'Connor, 1973; Offe, 1984).

None of this is to say that the state is the simple tool of capital envisaged in 'vulgar' or old-fashioned orthodox Marxism. According to the new left capitalist interests are divided, for example between industrial capital and finance capital, or between local capital and international capital. State policies cannot simply be 'read off' from the wishes expressed in the privacy of multinational boardrooms. The state is a force in its own right, as well as a battleground. But it can only manoeuvre within certain limits, or its economic underpinning will (without any need to posit a conscious 'capitalist plot') begin to collapse.

What, then, are the remedies that flow from this analysis? Here again the new left diverges sharply from the new right. The neo-Marxist analysis is a heavily *structuralist* perspective, whereas public choice theory is usually *individualist*. At the heart of the left's solution lies not the limiting of political and governmental activity prescribed by public choice theorists, but rather a radical *increase* in political participation. The new left has lost some of orthodox Marxism's scepticism concerning elections and representative democratic institutions. It wishes to see these strengthened and extended (as in proposals for health authority members to be directly elected rather than appointed - see, for instance Lowe, 1988). But, more important and radical than this, it has high hopes for the introduction of a variety of forms of *direct* democracy - particularly in the workplace and the local community (Held, 1987, pp.257–61). In such an increase in direct participation the new left see the seeds of the broader social transformation which their analysis claims is required. If the workers themselves have a major, direct say in controlling their own day-to-day conditions of work, the question of occupational health and safety will be accorded the prominence it has hitherto so often failed to achieve.

Few on the left believe such changes can be achieved quietly, through the 'normal' processes of élite accommodation described in the section on liberal corporatism. These élites are, in the neo-Marxist view, too deeply rooted in underlying class interests ever to be prepared to move voluntarily towards a radically more equal society. In such a society highly paid expertise such as that possessed by the medical profession would be made subject to full public accountability and responsive to widely established public health priorities. Major changes of this kind will only come after a period of class struggle during which sustained and organized pressure would have to be brought to bear on the existing power structure. Crisis and conflict, rather than planning and debate, are seen as the true authors of transformation.

Many millions of words have been expended critiquing Marxism, as many by Marxists themselves as by non-Marxists. One aspect of Marxism which remains clear, however, is that, in all its varieties, it aspires to be a theory of very broad scope. Of all social theories it is possibly the most ambitious, claiming to show how whole societies grow, change and sometimes tear themselves apart. Marxists have a strong sense of history, and of the interconnectedness of contemporary events with deep underlying trends, whether it be the rise of the middle classes, the internationalization of financial markets or the growth of the welfare state. This olympian vantage point does, however, mean that Marxist theories are usually not particularly interested in studying the micro factors in the policy process – the personalities, chance coincidences or regulatory details.

The coherence of Marxist thought has probably been declining over the past thirty years, partly because of the fresh, exploratory character of some neo-Marxist writing. Different thinkers within the Marxist camp now take very different positions on, for example, the autonomy of the state, the primacy of social class as an explanatory variable (relative, say, to race or gender), the viability of Marx's labour theory of value and the allegedly 'scientific' character of Marx's own writings. Nevertheless the basic emphasis on the importance of class divisions, on control over the means of economic production and on the subtle role of ideologies in shaping issues and agendas all continue to give a distinctive flavour to Marxist approaches (see Dunleavy and O'Leary, 1987, pp.203–70 for a taste of the complexity of neo-Marxist thought).

The empirical consistency of Marxist theory is extremely hard to assess. Of course there has been no shortage of false predictions in popular Marxist writings, though perhaps forecasts of the final crisis and collapse of capitalism are a shade less frequent now than they were in the past. More academic Marxism has usually been shy of predictions, indeed there has been a certain hesitancy about indulging in detailed empirical research at all. 'Empiricism' is a sin, or at least a naivety, in the Marxist canon, and most Marxist writers remain more comfortable with 'reading off' points of apparent correspondence between their macro-theoretical predictions about the conduct of the capitalist state and the actual behaviour of governments. Detailed empirical testing is rare, and it is therefore hard to judge how consistent Marxism is below the macro level of analysis.

Conclusion

In this first chapter we have explained the aims of the book and described our approach to explaining social and political phenomena. A description of 'foreground' NHS decisionmaking (the 'shared version') was then introduced and subjected to critique. An important part of the critique was that the 'shared version' did not go wide or deep enough to give a clear overall view of the dynamics of the health policy process. It was therefore necessary to introduce a selection of theoretical perspectives designed to afford precisely this broader, deeper understanding.

These theoretical perspectives will be revisited in the chapters which are to come. The book cannot cover every facet of health policy, but it will include the crucial issues of how health services are funded and distributed, what use is made of them, the roles of some occupational groups and how, if at all, their effectiveness, efficiency, equity and responsiveness are assessed.

There are two final points which should be borne in mind as the discussion moves into the rich details of the health policy process. The first is that this detail cannot be satisfactorily comprehended without a basic factual knowledge of the institutional make-up of the NHS. It is not the job of this book to provide extensive institutional descriptions, but we have included, as an annexe, an organization chart and some brief details, along with an outline of the proposals of *Working for Patients* and some references to other books.

The second point is cautionary. As we work with theory and evidence we are constantly reminded of the importance of keeping very clear about both the *scope* of our findings and the *conditions* under which they appear to hold. Thus, for example, when looking at funding in the next chapter you might decide that a neo-Marxist interpretation is rather convincing. But when it comes to the politics of medical careers in Chapter 4 an élitist perspective may seem more enlightening. Also much depends on the *level* one is working at (national financial flows or individual medical careers), and the best theoretical tools for one kind of topic at one level may prove relatively blunt for another. What exists as an unbudgeable constraint at one level (e.g. a cash limit for a District Health Authority) may be a matter of policy choice at another (the Treasury and the DoH may decide to inject more funds into the NHS). So at any given level the analyst needs carefully to specify the range of issues/relationships under consideration (scope) and the key conditions which appear to constrain them. This painstaking process can only be begun in the present volume. Even a limited effort, however, can soon dissolve many of the crude stereotypes and sweeping generalizations which so often bedevil discussion of our health services.

2 Funding health services

Introduction

The financing of health services both in the United Kingdom and in other developed countries is a constant source of lively debate. In recent years, the growth and control of expenditure on health care have been major concerns of all such countries. They remain vexing problems even for those countries which, like the United Kingdom, have managed to exert some degree of restraint on the rate of growth of the NHS. As an OECD report stated in 1985: 'All countries face a wide range of decisions about the management structure and financing of their health services' (OECD, 1985, p.9). Chapter 3 considers the changes in management and structure of the NHS over the past decade or so. In this chapter we are concerned with the basis of the funding of the NHS and with arguments that it is under-funded, and alternative sources of funding that have been canvassed over the years; finally we comment on the proposals for change in the 1989 White Paper which have a bearing on the future funding of the NHS. For further details concerning the White Paper, readers are referred to the Annexe.

The structure of the National Health Service, and its funding arrangements, are often seen as provoking controversy about whether health services are adequately funded or, as many both in and outside the NHS allege, under-funded. A former health minister, Enoch Powell, maintained that the centralized nature of NHS funding and public accountability encouraged a 'deafening chorus of complaint which rises day and night from every part of it' and 'a vested interest in denigration' among those working in it (Powell, 1976, p.16). There are, in addition, other forces at work creating pressures for more resources. There is always pressure for more resources because there are always new treatments to offer, or desirable modifications to existing practices to be sought. In the absence of agreed outcomes, resisting demands for more resources becomes problematic. In addition, since at least the late 1960s, real health spending has been climbing because of the combined influence of ageing populations and rapid technical progress. These pressures and others place a continual strain on the ability of governments to contain expenditure and maintain an optimal level of spending. As we show later, problems have arisen in the 1980s as a result of increased demand outstripping available resources.

Over the past decade, arguments over NHS funding have become more acute as a result of the Conservative administration's determination to control and contain public expenditure. Indeed, it was an alleged 'crisis' in NHS funding during the winter of 1986/87 that led the Prime Minister to set up a review of the Service. Paradoxically, the proposals for change which emerged from the review in the January 1989 White Paper, *Working for Patients* (Department of Health et al, 1989b) have virtually nothing to say about the actual *level* of funding of the NHS and very little on its source. The government remains committed to funding the NHS largely from general taxation while seeking to encourage people who can afford to do so to exit from the NHS in favour of private health care facilities. According to this view, pressure is eased on the NHS for those unable to obtain help elsewhere. Indeed, Mrs. Thatcher has let it be known that the NHS could only cater for those in real need if there was a flourishing private sector (Hunter, 1983a).

Financing the NHS

Public expenditure in the United Kingdom amounts to over 40 per cent of the gross domestic product (GDP). Within this percentage, central government's share is in the region of 75 per cent with local authorities being responsible for most of the remaining 25 per cent. The NHS receives most of its funds from general taxation (85 per cent in 1986/87) with the remainder coming from national insurance contributions (12 per cent) and prescription charges (3 per cent). The amount of expenditure from general taxation is agreed each year for the following three years through the Public Expenditure Survey (see Table 2.1).

Each summer the government considers its expenditure plans. This process takes the form of an examination of existing plans and an assessment of the scope and need for changes. Spending departments like the Department of Health review their spending plans to reflect the scope for further efficiencies and the need for additional development and expansion. The process proceeds in a series of negotiations between the spending departments and the Treasury within guidelines approved by ministers earlier in the year, which normally include an overall ceiling to total public expenditure. The Public Expenditure Survey Committee (PESC), an inter-departmental group of officials chaired by the Treasury,

Table 2.1 *Expenditure on UK health care as a percentage of GDP 1979–86*

Year	Total %	Net Public %	Private %
1979	5.2	4.7	0.5
1980	5.8	5.2	0.6
1981	6.0	5.4	0.6
1982	5.9	5.2	0.7
1983	6.1	5.4	0.7
1984	6.2	5.4	0.8
1985	6.0	5.2	0.8
1986	6.1	5.3	0.8

Source: The Directory of Independent Hospitals and Health Services 1988/89, Longman, 1988.

oversees and coordinates the process. Spending plans are finalized in the Chancellor of the Exchequer's autumn economic statement in November and this is published in more detail in a subsequent White Paper on public expenditure which describes the main features of the various spending plans within the context of the government's overall fiscal and economic policy. The NHS is not directly involved in the public expenditure survey but is represented by the Department of Health. However, health authorities can exert some influence over the process by ensuring that the Department is aware of current problems and financial difficulties. Much of this lobbying is conducted in public through the media and lies at the heart of Powell's misgivings about a process which offers every incentive to complain of deficiencies.

The funds made available for hospital and community health services are cash-limited unlike most of those available to family practitioner services (FPS), which are open-ended. This is shared out between the four countries making up the United Kingdom, with the health service allocation to Wales, Scotland and Northern Ireland forming part of the block grant which is then divided up by spending programme by the respective secretaries of state, who have discretion to allocate expenditure between individual authorities. Health authorities receive their allocations through the mechanism of a resource allocation formula, which is described in the next chapter. Once health authorities have been notified of their cash limits, they can begin to spend that money. Health authorities have revenue and capital cash limits, and in addition, may have earmarked revenue or capital allocations for specific purposes, such as joint finance for community care provision, waiting list initiatives, and AIDS. By far the biggest expense in the health service is the wages and salaries bill, which amounts to some 75 per cent of the total revenue cash limit. Other items of spending financed by the revenue cash limits include drugs, medical and surgical consumables, energy, transport costs, and so on.

Demand for health care

To meet new demands on services, the government estimates the necessary growth in expenditure for each year. This increase in resources in real terms is deemed necessary to meet the demands of demographic change, advances in medical technology and drug therapy, and service development. As part of its planning procedures, the Department of Health calculates the actual increase in expenditure that it estimates will be necessary each year to meet these extra requirements.

Perhaps the most important single demographic change is the increasing number of the very elderly, those of 75 years old and over. Table 2.2 indicates that their numbers, and proportion within the total population, will continue to grow until well into the next century.

Table 2.2 *The increasing numbers of the elderly*

Year	UK Population (millions)	75 Years and Over (millions)
1951	50.3	1.8
1961	52.8	2.4
1971	55.9	2.7
1981	56.4	3.3
1991	57.5	4.0
2001	59.0	4.4
2011	59.4	4.4

Source: *Social Trends*, no. 18, 1988.

Although this increase seems modest in number, its financial consequences are not. The average person over 75 consumes something like nine times the volume of health care resources used by the average person of working age, or five times the average for all ages (DHSS, 1983). Extrapolation of these proportions suggests that health authority budgets would need to increase in real terms by roughly one per cent *per annum* (Social Services Committee, 1986, p.xiii), a figure formally accepted by the government, though the matter is by no means uncontentious.

The method used by the Department to calculate demographic trends involves the following stages (King's Fund Institute, 1987):

- total hospital and community health services (HCHS) expenditure is apportioned to individual service categories, e.g. acute inpatient, outpatient, mental illness, mental handicap, geriatrics, etc;
- age-specific use rates for each service category – adjusted for higher degrees of 'dependency' of very young and elderly patients – are employed to allocate the total costs of each service by age group;
- total HCHS costs by age group are obtained by adding the age-specific costs for each service category;
- total HCHS costs incurred by each age group are divided by total population numbers in that group to obtain per capita expenditure; and
- per capita expenditure figures are combined with changes in total population numbers estimated by the OPCS to obtain the final estimates of total expenditure requirements.

Bosanquet (1985) has pointed to problems in the methodology used. In particular he is critical of the conservative nature of the basis of expenditure requirements since they relate to the total costs of treatment at *existing rates of treatment*. No allowance is made for improved performance or for new service developments which could affect service levels. Bosanquet also cites evidence to show that the sums of money allocated to the additional numbers of elderly people are not actually being spent on those services being used by this group.

In regard to medical advances, the DoH estimates that these absorb in the region of 0.5 per cent of resources annually (DHSS, 1983). Medical advances comprise the introduction of new technology and drug treatments. Although all new techniques need not always be more expensive – indeed, developments in day case surgery and endoscopy ought to reduce costs – many are. Whether such new advances are always efficient and efficacious in terms of their impact on health status is often impossible to say. (The problems of outcome measurement are discussed in Chapter 5.) Moreover, the figure of 0.5 per cent does not profess to represent what is *needed* or what is *feasible* medically. It is essentially a supply-side constrained figure which reflects public expenditure aims (and ultimately political values) more than health care considerations.

Resources for service development are intended to finance specific policy objectives determined by the DoH which it expects health authorities to pursue. In recent years priority had been attached to a number of developments, including combating the spread of AIDS, reducing waiting lists and waiting times, and developing heart surgery. This diverse and changing set of objectives amounts to a further 0.5 per cent additional demand each year. How well-founded the figure is in terms of the actual cost of policy developments is hard to say, but it seems likely that it is a somewhat arbitrary calculation (King's Fund Institute, 1987).

Whether expenditure overall has kept pace with increased demand as identified according to the three parameters just described − demographic change, medical advance and service development − is the subject of intense debate. According to the Social Services Committee, an increase in funding for the NHS of at least 2 per cent per year in real terms is required simply to maintain existing levels of revenue while keeping up with demographic and technological changes (Social Services Committee, 1988). The committee argues that this figure is accepted by the overwhelming majority of organizations representing health service staff. However, the DoH does not accept that an annual rise of 2 per cent is essential, preferring to place its faith in cost improvement programmes (CIPs) to generate greater efficiency. Available evidence suggests that during the 1980s expenditure on the NHS has not kept pace with increased demand (see Table 2.3). The table shows that since 1983 in only one year, 1987/88, has the annual increase in resources alone been sufficient to provide a substantial increase in real resources. The margins available for service development locally have indeed depended upon local CIPs.

The supply of resources

These tight constraints on health service finance owe a good deal to the economic crisis of the mid-1970s, when sharp increases in the price of oil caused severe contractions in the world economy. In the United Kingdom the then Labour government responded with a shift of emphasis from planning public expenditure in *volume* terms (in which cash spending is adjusted for changes in the prices of inputs within the health sector) to planning in *cash* terms (in which the cost of inputs is measured at the price levels current during the year in which the spending occurs), and a system of rigidly enforced cash limits, which offers greater control over expenditure levels. Previously, if the actual rate of inflation exceeded the expected rate, so that cash expenditure

Table 2.3 *Trends in Health Service purchasing power and margins for service development*

	HCHS Current % change in purchasing power	HCHS plus CIPs: margin for service development (%)	FPS % change in purchasing power
1979/80	0.1	0.1	0.4
1980/81	0.9	0.9	0.1
1981/82	2.0	2.0	2.0
1982/83	0.8	0.8	3.6
1983/84	0.0	0.0	2.0
1984/85	−0.1	1.0	2.8
1985/86	0.1	1.5	0.2
1986/87	0.5	2.0	2.5
1987/88	1.8	3.2	3.8
1988/89	0.4	1.8	4.1
TOTAL	6.5	13.3	21.5

Source: Social Services Committee, 1988, p.60.

overshot its target, cash shortfalls were made good in the following year.

Since 1979, this rigid control has been reinforced by the macro-economic policy of the Conservative government, which has been based on the view that the Public Sector Borrowing Requirement (PSBR) should comprise a declining proportion of GDP (Jackson, 1985), and indeed, more recently, that there should be no such PSBR. In a period of extremely modest economic growth, this has naturally placed great pressure on public expenditure, especially its cash-limited components, which, as we have seen, includes most of the NHS. (For a review see Harrison, 1988a; King's Fund Institute, 1988, pp.76–82.)

An obvious manifestation of this trend has been the falling rates of growth in real spending on health care. In the decade prior to 1974, the annual rate of increase in spending on HCHS after adjusting for general inflation was around 6 per cent annually whereas in the second half of the 1970s it grew at an average annual rate of less than 3 per cent (Judge, 1982). Despite rising overall levels of spending on HCHS during the 1980s, inflation has also taken its toll, since over the period the NHS has had to finance pay awards to staff and purchase the goods it uses. Measurement of inflation is an area of some debate, with the government preferring to use the GDP deflator to account for the inflation effect. This measures changes in prices in the economy as a whole, but it is argued that the inflationary pressures to which the NHS is subject differ from those represented by this measure. An alternative measure which is believed to reflect better the inflationary pressures on the NHS is the HCHS pay and prices deflator. This is based on movements in pay and prices directly relevant to health care (CIPFA, 1987).

Hence, much of the substantial additional cash allocated to the NHS during the 1980s has served only to compensate for rising rates of health service inflation. Despite a doubling of the cash increase in total spending on hospital and community health services from £500 million in 1985/86 6 to £1 billion in 1989/90, the increase in purchasing power (the development margin) has, as Table 2.3 shows, remained small. This limited margin for service development has coincided with a period of demographic change, as was shown in Table 2.2. It has been estimated that the funds needed to meet these would entail annual real increases of between 0.5 and one per cent during the 1990s.

The task of measuring the amount of additional finance which would have been required during this period is beset with technical and political difficulties. However, it has been estimated that by 1987/88 an extra £390 million would have been needed to re-establish the purchasing power expenditure level of 1981/82 (King's Fund Institute, 1988). Put another way, the Social Services Committee (1988, paragraph 12, viii) has estimated that after allowing for efficiency gains and cash-releasing cost improvements, the underfunding of the hospital and community health services between 1980/81 and 1987/88 was in the region of £1.5 billion at 1987/88 prices. In contrast to spending on HCHS, spending on FPS fared better with an annual growth during most of the 1980s of between 2.5 and 3 per cent. FPS, it will be recalled, are largely non cash-limited.

Although the NHS has been subjected to financial stringency, it has nevertheless fared better than most other areas of public expenditure. Only defence and social security expenditure have registered larger increases in real terms, the latter because it is largely *not* cash-limited. However, public opinion appears to remain unconvinced that the present level of expenditure on the NHS is sufficient. Repeated public opinion surveys show that the NHS is top of the public's list in terms of priorities for extra government spending (Taylor-Gooby, 1985).

A further issue of concern in terms of the financing of the NHS, but one which often goes unnoticed, is the difference in the funding levels between the four health services making up the United Kingdom. Spending on health services is significantly higher in Scotland, Wales and Northern Ireland than is the case in

Table 2.4 *Health Services expenditure in the UK: selected years*

	1979/80 Total £m	1979/80 Per capita £	1982/83 Total £m	1982/83 Per capita £	1985/86 Total £m	1985/86 Per capita £
England	7,341	158	11,426	244	13,932	296
Wales	462	167	738	263	891	317
Scotland	985	191	1,533	297	1,856	361
Northern Ireland	308	200	481	307	594	382

Source: Office of Health Economics, 1987.

England (see Table 2.4). Expenditure also varies between different regions and areas *within* each of the countries. Several observers have drawn attention to this apparent anomaly (Hunter, 1982 and 1983b; Birch and Maynard, 1986). The Social Services Committee (1989) returned to the issue in its examination of the White Paper, *Working for Patients*. In 1988/89 estimated gross public expenditure per head of population on health services in England was £390 compared with £425 in Wales, £430 in Northern Ireland and £485 in Scotland. As Table 2.4 shows, these striking differences in health expenditure levels have been an enduring feature of the NHS in the United Kingdom since its creation. Indeed, in their 1986 study Birch and Maynard confirmed that the differences between the four countries has widened since they first looked at the position in 1980. According to the Central Statistical Office (1986), Scotland accounts for a larger share of national expenditure than its population share while Wales accounts for a proportionate share.

These figures on expenditure make no allowance for differences in demand or need for health services nor for differences in the cost of delivering health care although these factors have been cited to account, in large part, for Scotland's generous share of resources. Similar arguments apply in Northern Ireland and, to a lesser extent, Wales where as in Scotland, there are a handful of dense urban areas and large tracts of sparsely populated rural hinterlands.

As the Social Services Committee's (1989) report makes clear, the present system of allocating resources according to separate formulae in each of the four countries (those operating in Wales, Scotland and Northern Ireland are variants of the RAWP formula in England) does not make explicit the differences in levels of expenditure. The proposal in the White Paper, *Working for Patients*, to allocate resources on a capitation basis will do so. In this way, it will be possible to demonstrate that in each of the four countries funding is clearly related to need. The capitation basis of resource allocation will be weighted to reflect the health and age distribution of the population, including the number of elderly people, and the relative costs of providing services (Department of Health et al, 1989b, para. 4.8).

Under-funding

The question of whether or not the NHS is under-funded is not easy to answer in unequivocal or objective terms. There is no 'right level' of spending on health care, and as events have proved, no finite amount of ill health despite the illusions of the NHS's architects. Need and demand are not absolute states but elastic concepts. The ability to consume health care resources is apparently limitless. We have seen that needs and demands are potentially infinite or highly elastic as people's expectations change, as populations age and people live longer, and as new drugs and medical techniques are developed which require – and create pressure for – additional resources. In most, though not all, cases they have created a need or demand where formerly there was none. Good examples are the growth of bioengineering, and the development of artificial joints (e.g. replacement hips), arteries, heart valves, and so on.

International comparisons suggest that although the NHS may be near the bottom of the league in terms of the proportion of gross national product devoted to health services, there is no firm evidence that the United Kingdom is less healthy or, to put it another way, that greater expenditure automatically leads to better health (see Table 2.5). As the Royal Commission on the NHS pointed out: 'It is at least arguable that the improvement in the health of the nation would be greater if extra resources were, for example, devoted to better housing' (1979, p.334). There is also a further argument concerning whether existing resources are being used to their maximum benefit. According to this view, under-funding is not the main problem with the NHS; rather it is one of securing the desired outcomes from a given input of resources and avoiding counterproductive results. The issue, therefore, is one of the efficient and effective use of resources, rather than their overall level. Indeed, this view has been the linchpin of government policy towards the NHS over the past decade and, as we discuss in Chapter 3, underlines a series of management reforms designed to improve efficiency in resource use.

As Allsop (1984, p.80) points out, 'arguments about levels of

Table 2.5 *Health expenditure: international comparisons as a percentage of GDP, 1984*

Country	% GDP
Australia	7.8
Denmark	6.3
France	9.1
West Germany	8.1
Greece	4.6
Italy	7.2
Japan	6.6
Netherlands	8.6
Spain	5.8
Sweden	9.4
UK	5.9
USA	10.7
Average	7.2

Source: OECD, 1987.

funding are largely meaningless' precisely because they say little about the efficiency of that spending. Historically, most advanced economies' expenditures on health have tended to grow in line with increases in wealth. As long as the United Kingdom economy remains fairly stagnant, it is unlikely that the NHS's share of spending will grow markedly unless there is a dramatic shift in public spending priorities. As Lee (1982, p.75) argues: 'There is no precise calculus for determining the priority for health services as against other programmes of public expenditure.' Even if a wide measure of agreement exists that expenditure on health services should increase, support also exists for increases in other policy sectors like education, transport and, more recently, the environment generally, which embraces much public health activity. However, even allowing for these factors, *per capita* spending in the United Kingdom is nearly 30 per cent below the level that would be expected in terms of the United Kingdom's gross domestic product per head (King's Fund Institute, 1988). The figures show that the United Kingdom not only spends less than expected in terms of private expenditure but also that public expenditure is approximately 10 per cent below its expected level. Put another way, even if private funding of health care were to increase, international evidence still suggests that public expenditure is up to £2 billion below its expected level in the United Kingdom.

Despite the persistence of a general state of excess demand over supply there do seem to be some special circumstances surrounding the experience of the 1980s (King's Fund Institute, 1988). These relate to both the demand and supply of health care and were noted earlier. On the demand side, two factors distinguish the period. First, there has been substantial growth in the size of the elderly population, especially in the numbers of very elderly people (i.e. those aged 85 and over whose numbers will show an increase of 32 per cent from 1988 to 1995 : OPCS, 1987). Second, there have been rising public expectations. It has been suggested that people's expectations of health care provision are increasing at an exponential rate and that this is producing a widening gap between expectations and NHS service levels (Thwaites, 1987). Certainly, international studies suggest that in those countries where people are able to choose the amount that they spend on health care, the share of their income so spent increases as their income rises. The subject of expectations is a complex one. It does appear that the case for an *acceleration* in the rate of growth of expectations is not proven. If there is a problem in connection with expectations, it centres more on the failure of supply to match steadily increasing demand. The supply problems of the 1980s centre on three main issues: tightening public expenditure constraints; the privatization programme; and the scope for greater efficiency in the use of NHS resources. We have already commented on the first of these issues; the other two are considered later in this chapter.

At the end of the day, whether the NHS is under-funded or receives a level of funding that is about right is an impossible question to answer. As we have intimated, the argument about under-funding is complex and inconclusive. Those with a vested interest in seeing services grow and expand will side with those who support the under-funding thesis. On the other side are ranged those who maintain that unless it can be demonstrated beyond reasonable doubt that minimum standards of care are being eroded, there exists no sound evidence to support regular additional massive injections of resources. Ultimately, it is a political issue. The *economist's* view is that until we know the costs and (more importantly) the benefits arising from different categories of expenditure it is impossible to say whether present levels of aggregate funding are too low, too high, or are at the optimal level. To enable rational resource allocation decisions to be made, far more information is required about the relationship between health care inputs and health status outputs/outcomes.

The *needs* approach is a method utilizing the best available estimates of the growth in health care needs in order to determine the extra funds that the NHS will require to meet them each year. As we mentioned earlier, growth of needs derives from three main sources: demographic change, medical advance, and nationally determined service priorities. There are considerable methodological problems associated with the way in which these estimates are produced (Harrison and Gretton, 1986) but the Department of Health has accepted them as a quantified statement of what would be required to meet the additional demands being placed on the health service. In this sense they at least provide a benchmark for assessing public expenditure levels even if their validity is in some doubt.

A third approach to the question of funding levels has been outlined in a report from the Institute of Health Services Management published in 1987 (O'Higgins, 1987). In an attempt to depoliticize the issue of funding for health care services, the report suggested that a minimum consensus should be sought that would provide a basis for planning the growth of health expenditure for at least the duration of the present Parliament. To achieve this aim, the report proposed moving away from the demand or needs approach to one in which the growth in health care expenditure would be based upon what the country could afford. Thus, the report proposed that health care spending should, as a minimum, rise in line with national income. In addition, it argued that this rate for growth would need to be augmented with separate provision for such factors as demographic change, major new service needs and any possible pay restructuring resulting from, for example, the need to attract more nurses into the NHS.

Sources of funds

As we have stated, by far the major source of funding in respect of the NHS is general taxation. This makes the NHS a near monopoly public service largely financed from public expenditure which is under direct political control in the shape of the Secretary of State for Health, who is accountable to Parliament for the running of the NHS. In the view of (among others) a former permanent secretary at the Department of Health, Sir Kenneth Stowe, as long as Parliament votes the vast sums of money spent on the NHS (£27 billion in 1989) it will always be the case that limits will be placed on the extent to which health authorities at the periphery will be able to exercise discretion over the way in which those funds are spent. In Stowe's words: (1989, p.55) 'The key to the future development of our health care system – its scope, structure, finance, and functioning in every respect . . . lies in my view in the definition of the role of Parliament.'

The funding mechanism underpinning the NHS is a deliberate social and political act which reflects a political decision about the nature of health, health services, and society's role in providing them. The basis of the funding of the NHS is a belief in equality of access to health care services according to need and not ability to pay. Health care, it is argued, is a fundamental human right which should be free at the point of use with no financial barriers impeding access. Prescription charges have eroded this principle and tax relief on health insurance for the over 60s – as proposed in the 1989 White Paper – will erode it further, but it remains largely intact and is the pillar upon which the NHS was established.

Over the last decade or so there have been attempts to look for other sources of funding such as insurance schemes and an enlarged private health care sector. The search has not hitherto led to any major shift in policy. Operating separately from the NHS, but with clear implications for public provision, is a sizeable private health care sector, though still small by comparison with the NHS. Before considering the private independent sector in more detail we first look at proposals for supplementary finance and insurance funding.

Supplementary finance

Supplementary funding is probably the least contentious of all the alternative sources of finance, for it seeks not to disturb in a fundamental way the established basis of the NHS but rather to augment it with funds from other sources. One such source is charges to patients at the time they use particular services. Prescription charges fall into this category. Charges for 'hotel' services (e.g. accommodation, meals and so on) have been considered from time to time but have been ruled out on grounds of administrative cost since there would have to be exemptions for those patients below a specified income.

A second possible source of supplementary funding is hypothecation, that is, the earmarking of particular taxes or contributions specifically for use in the NHS. National Insurance contributions come into this category but, as we have seen, they account for a minimal proportion of NHS finance. A case has been made for introducing hypothecated taxes on the sale of harmful goods such as alcohol and tobacco products (King's Fund, 1988). The problem with hypothecation is that governments generally dislike earmarking taxes for particular purposes since it reduces their freedom to allocate expenditure.

A third possible source of supplementary finance is the organization of lotteries, bazaars, appeals, jumble sales and so on. All of these have at one time or another appeared on the NHS landscape either nationally or at a local level. However, their contribution to the overall funds available to the NHS has been marginal and is likely to remain so. Moreover, the yield from such initiatives tends to be uncertain and expensive to administer, thereby reducing their efficiency and appeal.

A fourth approach which represents an indirect form of supplementary finance has been the cost improvement programmes (CIPs) in the NHS which were introduced in 1984/85. Health authorities have been expected to deliver at least 1 per cent of their cash allocations each year in cash releasing CIPs. DHSS guidance to health authorities defines cost improvements as:

> Measures which are aimed at releasing cash or manpower used in providing a service by getting the same service output for a smaller input of resources; or improving productivity by getting a higher output for the same input (or a less than proportionate increase in input) (quoted in National Audit Office, 1986, para. 2.8).

Health authorities have been obliged by central government to use these programmes as a minor source of funds for service development. In 1988/89 they were expected to produce an additional £900 million through cash releasing savings. However, the National Audit Office (1986) in monitoring these programmes pointed to the potential dangers of reductions in the quality of service and alluded to the prospects of diminishing returns in this area. Moreover, as the NAO asserted, it is not always easy to distinguish a cost improvement from an actual cut in service. The NAO concluded:

> At some DHAs there was evidence that the focus was on saving costs without necessarily any matching improvement in efficiency. For example, some emphasis had been on setting lower budgets and expecting individual managers to remain within them. In such cases it was not always clear whether savings had been made without corresponding reductions in the standards of health care provided (NAO, 1986, para. 2.15).

These concerns have been reaffirmed more recently in a joint study by the IHSM, King's Fund Institute and NAHA (King's Fund Institute, 1989).

A further source of supplementary funding in recent years has been income generation from non-clinical activities. Many hospitals have developed commercial activities, mainly in their concourse and waiting areas. These include: cafeteria services; newspaper stalls and bookshops; food shops; florists; hairdressers; chemists; photography concessions in maternity hospitals; taxi phone lines; leasing advertising space; installing video entertainment systems, and so on. In some health districts more ambitious schemes have been considered, including extending services outside the NHS, such as bidding for school catering contracts. The Department of Health has established a unit with special responsibility for income generation, and the 1988 Health and Medicines Act opened up possibilities for greater income-generating activity.

The main reservations surrounding income generation schemes centre on two issues: are they worthwhile given the levels of income they attract? And do they detract from management's main task of improving patient care by running health services? On the first question it does seem to be the case that the sums that can be raised are rather small. A report by the Scottish Health Service Management Efficiency Group (1987) suggested that there was scope for raising just under £2 million per year in Scotland but this compares with a total hospital and community health services revenue budget of £1,300 million. In England it has been suggested that up to £135 million per year could be raised in the long term. But even this represents only just over 1 per cent of the current hospital and community health service revenue budget. On the other hand, such sums of money, small though they may be, should not be dismissed in a period of very tight funding. However, there is an issue concerning the amount of management time taken up by such activities and whether or not it amounts to a serious distraction from the business of actually running and providing health services. Clearly, income generation is an activity for marketing managers rather than for health service managers.

An indirect source of additional finance, and usually included in the CIPs but with separate consideration, is the competitive tendering initiative for the supply of domestic, laundry and catering services between health authorities' in-house direct labour services and private external contractors. Health authorities spend over £1,000 million a year on the 'hotel' functions. By making contracts for such services subject to competition with private firms the government believes that savings will be available for retention by health authorities for use in developing services. Approximately 85 per cent of contracts have been awarded in-house (NAHA, 1989, para. 9, p.187). Since 1982 the number of directly employed ancillary staff has fallen by 30 per cent (NAHA, 1989, para. 22, p.174). Whether standards have been maintained, improved, or have fallen is arguable. Certainly anecdotal evidence abounds concerning dirty floors and laundry and increased pressure on staff who often work longer shifts and/or have heavier workloads. We discuss this further in Chapter 4.

Finally, health voucher schemes are sometimes seen as a means of attracting additional finance into health care. In fact they are more a method of deploying a given public spending allocation in a way that gives greater power to consumers. In essence, such a scheme would involve allocating a voucher of a fixed nominal value to every individual with which he or she could buy health services of choice. In this way, it is argued, consumer choice would be enhanced; at least minimum levels of treatment would be guaranteed to all; and competition for business between suppliers would act as a spur to greater efficiency. Additional finance would be forthcoming to the extent that people wished to top up their voucher with private expenditure.

An NHS voucher scheme has been introduced for spectacles but this is a relatively straightforward market. Elsewhere, vouchers have been widely discussed in connection with education, but limited demonstrations of schemes and feasibility studies have revealed serious difficulties with them. This does not augur well for the considerably more complex health sector. In particular there is the major problem posed by extreme variations in demand for health care. The average *per capita* public expenditure of approximately £375 has been cited as a basis for nominal value of the voucher. Although this would be sufficient for low-risk groups to purchase private health insurance, it would obviously not cover adequately actuarially based premium payments required from high-risk groups. Advocates for the voucher profess to recognize this problem and suggest 'community rating' among various population groups, i.e. the young, the elderly, and so on, so that voucher values compensate poor risks (Goldsmith, 1988). But even this refinement is unlikely to be able to take account of the substantial variations in demand within specific community rated groups. In short, vouchers are suited to those markets where there is relatively equal and homogeneous demand from all consumers. Since this does not apply in health care the results would include all the familiar problems of adverse selection.

Social insurance

The main alternative to financing the NHS out of central taxation is to do so through a health insurance scheme on the model of Western Europe or North America. The Royal Commission on the NHS in 1979 considered the advantages and disadvantages of insurance-based schemes, while acknowledging that there is no standard system of health insurance and that schemes have grown up over many years and reflect the peculiarities of the countries they serve.

The Commission pointed to two main disadvantages which arise in most insurance-based schemes: the fact that those groups in the community who are both bad health risks and too poor to pay high premiums (e.g. elderly people, children and mentally and physically handicapped people, who account for over sixty per cent of NHS spending) do not fare well; and the high cost of administration in order to collect funds. These reasons led the Commission to reject a switch to health insurance as the means of funding the NHS. Even partial insurance financing was regarded as problematic for it would carry the danger of producing a two tier system of health care. The present government has fewer reservations about such an outcome and believes (publicly at any rate) that any expansion of the private health insurance sector can only be beneficial to the NHS by easing pressures on it (Hunter, 1983a).

Private health insurance

Paying for health care, *planning* it and *providing* it are three separate activities, each of which may be organized through private or public institutions or some mixture of the two. In this section and the next section we consider the role of the private sector in these activities.

Ministers have pointed to low levels of private spending on health as an explanation of low levels of total health expenditure in the United Kingdom compared with most other OECD countries. In fact, as we noted earlier, part of the explanation lies in the lower level of public spending on health care provision in addition to the shortfall in private spending. Any major increase in private spending in the United Kingdom would probably depend on the growth of private health insurance. Most of this activity is likely also to involve an expansion of the growth of private supply at the expense of the NHS.

A key factor in the development of the private sector, which the government seeks to encourage, has been the spread of private medical insurance. It is the main engine of growth for private acute health care, about 70 per cent of which is claimed to be insurance-funded (NAHA, 1989, para. 4, p.43). Since 1979 the percentage of the population covered by some form of private health insurance has doubled, from under 5 per cent to 10 per cent.

In 1950, the number of people with private health care insurance fell to 50,000. At the end of 1987 an estimated 5.2 million people were covered by some form of it. This was a 6.7 per cent more than at the end of 1986, a figure which represents a significant acceleration of the growth rate of about 3 per cent per annum or less which took place throughout the early and mid-1980s. Whether public perceptions of the NHS account for this growth is difficult to say, although it does, as we have seen, correspond to a tightening fiscal squeeze on the NHS and growing media coverage of waiting lists and times, alleged resource shortages, and problems over standards of care.

About one half of private insurance is paid for by companies who offer it to their employees as part of their conditions of service. Such company-financed insurance has grown rapidly in recent years and is expected to continue to do so in the future. A key disadvantage with such private cover is that in most cases it stops when an individual retires. In a modest attempt to stimulate private insurance cover for retired persons the government has decided as part of the 1989 White Paper package to encourage its take-up. Legislation will be introduced from April 1990 to give income tax relief on premiums for those aged 60 and over, whether paid by them or by their families on their behalf (Department of Health et al, 1989b). As was noted earlier, this development breaches one of the fundamental principles of the NHS whereby services are available to all regardless of ability to pay. There are many, including some Conservative MPs, who believe that this particular proposal could be seen as the thin end of the wedge whereby the funding for health care shifts progressively from public funding in its entirety to a system where a proportion of funding comes from private sources.

Health ministers have made no secret of their desire to encourage private spending on health. It is a major plank in their policy for the provision of health care in the United Kingdom. As part of this policy, greater emphasis is likely to be placed upon private health insurance. International evidence suggests that where private insurance is the main form of health finance it has a number of failings. Adverse selection means that high-risk groups find it difficult to obtain cover at affordable premiums. Most policies exclude cover for catastrophic and long term, chronic illness. Insufficient control over treatment levels and prices has sometimes led to serious cost inflation and over-treatment for some conditions. Low-income households can rarely afford adequate cover. To meet these failings, in all advanced countries, governments have invariably assumed major responsibilities for finance. Even in the United States, over 40 per cent of total health expenditure is publicly financed (OECD, 1987).

In the early 1980s in the United Kingdom there was much talk of dismantling the NHS and replacing it with a private health insurance scheme. Following a report commissioned by the then Secretary of State for Social Services, which was never published, the proposal was shelved (Harrison, 1988a, pp.77–8) but it continues to surface from time to time as concern about the mounting cost of the NHS and the alleged deterioration of its fabric has continued to grow. However, as the 1989 White Paper makes clear, proposals for an extension of private health insurance no longer envisage it as a replacement for public finance. Rather it is seen as a source of supplementary or top-up finance.

The independent sector

When it reported some ten years ago, the Royal Commission on the NHS (1979, para. 18.41) felt able to conclude that 'It is clear that the private sector is too small to make a significant impact on the NHS, except locally and temporarily.' Such a statement no longer reflects the position of the private health care sector in the United Kingdom. This sector in 1987 supplied 10.7 per cent of all United Kingdom hospital-based treatment and cares compared with an estimated 9.6 per cent in 1986 and 7.5 per cent in 1984; independent health care supply amounted to an estimated £4.4 million in 1987 – an 18 per cent increase on 1986 (Laing, 1988). In 1979, when the Royal Commission reported, under 5 per cent of the population was covered by private health insurance provided by the three principal provident associations, and the benefits paid out represented less than 1 per cent of NHS expenditure (Office of Health Economics, 1987). But, even then, this general picture was misleading because it masked the importance of the private sector in particular geographical areas and specialties. For example, Nicholl and others (1984) showed that in 1981 the combined private sector in England and Wales accounted for 13.2 per cent of total caseload in domestic, inpatient elective surgery. Within this surgical category, the private sector performed over 20 per cent of haemorrhoidectomies, hysterectomies, total hip replacements and procedures for ligation and stripping of varicose veins.

However, it is the rate of growth of private finance and provision during the 1980s that has changed the picture quite dramatically. The most rapid growth in provision has occurred in nursing and residential care homes for elderly people. In this case, much of the expansion has been fuelled by the ready availability of public finances through the social security system (Audit Commission, 1986; National Audit Office, 1987). But as far as the acute sector is concerned, data analysed by the Sheffield Medical Care Research Unit suggest that there was also a marked increase in activity between 1981 and 1986 (Williams, 1987). This is the changed context within which the private sector must be examined at the close of the 1980s.

Table 2.6 *UK independent hospitals: ownership 1979 and 1986*

Category	1979 No. of Hospitals	1979 No. of Beds	1979 % of Total	1986 No. of Hospitals	1986 No. of Beds	1986 % of Total
Charitable						
Religious	33	1,940	29.0	23	1,420	14.2
Charitable	22	1,686	25.2	29	1,991	19.9
Charitable Groups	33	1,149	17.2	37	1,436	14.3
Charitable Total	88	4,775	71.4	89	4,847	48.3
For-Profit						
American Groups	3	366	5.5	31	2,239	22.3
British Groups	4	156	2.3	35	1,535	15.3
Independent	55	1,394	20.8	43	1,404	14.0
For-Profit Total	62	1,916	28.6	109	5,178	51.7

Source: Laing's Review of Private Healthcare 1987, Laing and Buisson, 1987.

The private acute sector comprises both for-profit hospital and clinics and not-for-profit charitable institutions such as Nuffield Hospitals (see Table 2.6). In recent years growth has been more pronounced in the for-profit than the not-for-profit sector. The marked growth in private health insurance and increased activity within independent health care generally suggest that it is meeting an expanding source of consumer demand. In common with other systems of market allocation, the private finance and supply of health care offers a direct link between what people are willing to pay for and the service they receive. Subject to reservations (not always explicitly acknowledged) about the amount of information possessed by consumers of health care (mainly lack of expertise on medical matters), the advocates of such a system maintain that it is responsive to consumer preferences. Certainly consumers of private non-urgent acute care generally have access to services with a shorter waiting time than NHS patients and often enjoy higher standards of hotel services. But it is still only a small minority of the population who have access to these services. Even with the continued expansion of the private sector in the future this is almost certain to remain the case. It will act as a supplement to mainstream NHS services for certain relatively privileged groups of people and procedures.

In *Working for Patients*, the government asserts the NHS will continue to be financed mainly out of general taxation. Nevertheless, a growing role is favoured for the independent sector. According to the White Paper, the advantages brought about by the independent sector are that it increases the range of options available to patients, contributes to the cost-effective treatment of NHS patients, and responds flexibly and rapidly to patients' needs. The government is keen that these alleged advantages should be developed further. Whatever the ideological underpinnings of such a view, the government asserts that there are practical advantages too. In particular, it believes that a thriving independent sector relieves pressure on the NHS and increases opportunities for the NHS and the private sector to learn from each other and to support each other. Many of the White Paper's proposals are intended to open further opportunities for the two sectors to work together.

The government has pointed to the growing interdependence between the two sectors during the 1980s. For example, in 1986 contractual arrangements between the NHS and the private sector led to over 26,000 inpatient treatments at a cost of some £45 million. As part of the government's drive to reduce hospital waiting lists, many health authorities have entered into short-term contracts with private hospitals specifically to treat waiting list cases. The government wishes to build on these initiatives and believes that there is considerable scope for doing so. The intention is that GPs, for example, should be able to use NHS funds to pay for treatment in the private sector for certain conditions if this offers better quality or better value for money than buying NHS services. Similarly, health authorities as purchasers rather than providers of care will be free to buy in services from the private sector if it offers a better deal than is available from NHS hospitals. (See Annexe for further details.)

The reasons for the growth of the independent health care

sector are complex. Continuing financial stringency is a key factor behind the growth, together with public uncertainty and concern over NHS facilities in particular parts of the country. Collaborative activity between the public and private health care sectors has also been actively encouraged and has begun to develop rapidly. Perhaps too, a management culture more supportive of dealing with private sector providers has begun to spread through the NHS. Legislative and administrative barriers to joint ventures are being removed; the 1988 Health and Medicines Act, for example, opens up a number of possibilities for public–private partnership; moves towards an internal market as proposed in the 1989 White Paper could further encourage public–private health care trading activities. Once agreed pricing mechanisms are in place within the NHS, trading could be extended beyond the NHS to include independent health care suppliers.

An assessment

It is important to keep a sense of perspective on the developments in funding health care services reviewed in this chapter. For instance talk of massive growth in private health care developments is probably unnecessarily alarmist. Some sort of public–private mix is likely to remain a feature of health care provision, certainly as long as it is positively encouraged by central government. But the growth of the private sector has been uneven across the United Kingdom. There are large tracts of the country where its presence is minimal or non-existent and its impact on the public sector marginal. It is only in areas like London and the South East of England, and in major conurbations like Birmingham and Manchester, where private practice has flourished in recent years.

Although a shift to an insurance-based system has been ruled out on grounds of costs, the development of a two tier health care system is a distinct possibility in some parts of the country. Indeed, some observers would argue that it already exists (Griffith and Rayner, 1985). Under this scenario, the NHS will assume the role of a 'safety net' for the poor and others unable to obtain private cover. In this respect, it may be argued that the private sector will grow at the expense of the NHS. It is also the case that a thriving private sector may distort NHS priorities, as consultants, nurses, and other health care workers are attracted towards those specialties and parts of the countries where they can increase their income. A more optimistic scenario is that a partnership between the two sectors can only benefit the patient and improve services. This, at any rate, is what the government believes. What the private sector can offer, in their view, is flexibility, and the ability to change rapidly the amount of a particular service. For example, unacceptably long waiting times for hip replacements can be reduced.

If a mixed health economy is emerging in the United Kingdom in which the NHS will be by far the bigger partner, Maynard (1984, p.1851) may still be right in his view that:

> Private practice can never be an answer or an irrelevance. It will continue to frustrate socialists and liberals alike. The former would like its abolition and the latter its triumph, but such ideals are unattainable and the reality is that the problems facing the managers of the private sector are remarkably like those facing the managers of the NHS – cost containment, value for money – that is efficiency in the use of society's scarce resources.

No health care system anywhere is perfect or can meet all demands placed upon it, although some arrangements may be more successful than others in grappling with this dilemma. The NHS is no exception. The challenge confronting policymakers is to seek ways of reducing imperfections. Ultimately, a political choice has to be made in selecting the funding option – or options – most likely to secure the desired ends.

Funding: a theoretical explanation

Of the four theoretical perspectives reviewed in Chapter 1, our account of funding health services in the United Kingdom can best be explained by a combination of neo-élitist, neo-Marxist and public choice theories, although the last of these possesses less explanatory power than the others. Neo-pluralism is the weakest of all our theoretical approaches in its ability to explain the events reviewed in this chapter, though it cannot be entirely discounted.

All countries in the developed world operate health care systems which display a mix of public and private inputs in terms of their funding, planning and provision (Maxwell, 1981; Klein, 1982a). The United Kingdom is no exception and recent developments and proposals for reform, notably those contained in the 1989 White Paper, are designed to encourage a more pluralistic service delivery system which is separate from the funding of care. These developments are still in the embryonic stages and may remain essentially peripheral to the future of the

NHS. However, during the period covered by this book, the NHS has remained a near-monopoly public service. This 'steady state' requires an explanation, particularly at a time when few areas of public sector activity have escaped attack from a reforming government committed to a 'public choice' ideology. It is only in the last year or two that the NHS has come under close scrutiny from reformers.

In accounting for recent reform moves in the NHS, the prescriptive aspects of public choice theories do contribute to a better understanding, since the proposals are inspired by the new right's critique of inflexible, insensitive and public bureaucracies of which the NHS represents one of the few remaining, but seemingly the most resilient, examples. The assertion at the heart of the 1989 White Paper that more funding for the NHS is not the solution to the alleged crisis in health care can be accounted for by a public choice emphasis on the need to control and reduce public expenditure. In addition, the stress on value for money and CIPs is a manifestation of the public choice theorist's stress on maximizing the efficiency with which any resource is deployed. Many of the initiatives, such as CIPs and the search for new sources of finance, which have been a feature of funding policy since the mid-1980s, owe their origins to public choice concepts. However, to date these developments are of marginal significance as far as the total budget of the NHS is concerned.

We turn next to the neo-pluralist perspective since it can offer an explanation for the increasing incursion by big business and corporate interests into private health care in the United Kingdom. Until the last few years, the private sector in the United Kingdom comprised principally independent providers such as Nuffield Hospitals who were chiefly of a not-for-profit nature. With the expansion of private health care and its active encouragement by the government, this sector has begun to be transformed and be dominated by large American companies such as AMI, Humana, Hospital Corporation of America and others (Higgins, 1988). Still, however, the size of this sector is limited and leaves the vast public funding of the NHS and its evolution over the years to be explained. Thus, neither public choice nor neo-pluralistic approaches take us very far in this endeavour.

A neo-élitist perspective can be regarded as shedding light on the NHS's origins as an example of élite accommodation. The creation of the NHS as part of the emerging post-war welfare state consensus owes much to a pragmatic concern among corporate interests to maintain the existing social order. According to a neo-Marxist view, the state has been captured by capitalist interests. Neo-Marxists point to both the internationalization of capital and the particular connections between the Conservative party and the catering, cleaning, laundry and building industries to explain some of the policy developments of the 1980s such as competitive tendering involving the contracting out of various hotel services. Neo-Marxists would challenge public choice theorists' explanations for these developments (see above) and would argue that the broader socio-economic context and its shifting dynamics during the 1970s and 1980s cannot be ignored. In particular, the economic crises of the mid-1970s and early 1980s led capitalist states to 'roll back the frontiers of the welfare state' in order to create room for revived private profits. The economic strategy of the Thatcher government has been to reduce the tax burden on individuals thereby creating incentives to produce more private profits. Neo-élitist theories can best explain developments in health care spending over the years, and perhaps also the constraints that appear to be preventing the government making as rapid progress in the restructuring of the NHS as many of its most ardent new right supporters would like. Whereas public choice theorists are unable to explain success in holding down public expenditure on health care, neo-élitist theories are able to do so. The accommodation between élites in government and in the key provider group (the medical profession) has enabled tight control over spending to be maintained. This has not prevented the professions from complaining over the years that insufficient resources have been made available, but such discontent was containable during the first thirty years or so of the NHS. It has become more acute over the past decade as the government has strained to breaking point the accommodation or concordat with the medical profession, not merely over spending, but also over the latter's ability to practise medicine as it sees appropriate and to maintain its freedoms to allocate resources and make decisions about appropriate treatments. But while relations between the élite actors may be becoming strained, it is nevertheless the case that the NHS has been remarkably successful in maintaining its favourable funding position in the league table of public expenditure commitments. As we showed earlier, apart from a slight dip in the early 1980s, the NHS has successfully maintained a steady year-on-year incremental growth. Whether the growth has been sufficient to cover rising demands generated by new developments and demographic trends and to compensate for pay awards and inflation are matters for debate. But it cannot be denied that the élite consensus underpinning the NHS has remained remarkably robust. It would appear that in the health care sector, the élite triangle (i.e. the Whitehall–Westminster axis between civil servants and politicians, the higher echelons of the medical profession, and managers) has proven much more stubbornly resistant than in other areas of public policy such as housing, transport and education. Part of the explanation may lie in the special relationship not only between the NHS and the public but also between the medical profession and the public. (We discuss this further in Chapter 5.) It is qualitatively different from that in other sectors and may act as a brake on what the government would like to do as distinct from what it *can* do. The debate on funding is caught between public choice ideas on the one hand and neo-élitist thinking on the other, and remains unresolved.

Thus, a neo-élitist perspective helps account for the failure so far to shift significantly the funding base of the NHS. The reforms set out in *Working for Patients* (and described in the Annexe), stop far short of what the public choice theorists have advocated, although they can be seen as a softening up process in readiness for further changes in the same direction. Neo-Marxists would probably subscribe to this view for the reasons cited earlier. Nevertheless, arguably limitations on what would be acceptable to key groups, such as the medical profession, may have contributed to the move not so much to a full-blooded market economy of health but to a more mixed economy. Judging from the vociferous opposition to the White Paper proposals from virtually all provider groups, they may still be unacceptable to most of the relevant élites. Élite accommodation has, temporarily at least, broken down. For public choice theorists, the opposition is a clear reflection of the vested interests having their comfortable and protected lifestyles threatened. Such shroud-waving tactics are entirely predictable and in keeping with the new right's critique of public monopolies.

Finally, a neo-élitist perspective is helpful in explaining the persistence of intra-UK differences in levels of expenditure between the four countries. Whatever the reasons offered in terms of greater health needs accounting for the differences (see Hunter and Wistow, 1987) the figures do seem somewhat arbitrary and a consequence (possibly) of various interests seeking to maintain their advantage in the spending league table. Indeed, public choice theorists would argue that these differences in funding levels within the United Kingdom are a good example of budget maximization on the part of bureaucrats and providers. Similar assumptions underlie Powell's (1976) observation that it is in the interests of such groups always to denigrate the NHS in the hope of obtaining more resources. However, neo-élite theory concerning élite accommodation is probably a more persuasive explanation of intra-United Kingdom funding differences.

In summary then, no single theoretical approach will suffice to explain the pattern of NHS funding. Moreover, the explanatory power of the approaches we have been concerned with varies according to the period under discussion. Up until the 1980s, neo-élitist theories would have been most powerful. However, over the past decade or so, neo-Marxist explanations have acquired additional weight and public choice theories a greater prominence in seeking to explain policy developments on the other. Of the four theoretical perspectives we have employed, neo-pluralism has least to offer, but cannot be discounted entirely. Apart from explaining the greater penetration of big business into the United Kingdom health care market, continuing high public support for the NHS can be seen as a constraining factor on the government's ability to cut further public spending on health care, and its determination to subject the NHS to market forces as set out in the 1989 White Paper proposals. However, despite the possibility of lost support being translated into lost votes and even lost parliamentary seats, the government's public stance has been to ignore public opinion and to attempt to demonstrate that professional interests have deliberately sought to distort the proposals as a ploy to cause unjustified concern and alarm among vulnerable groups who, far from having anything to fear from the changes, have a great deal to gain (Harrison, 1990).

The recent history of funding policy in the NHS can be seen as a series of struggles and eventual trade-offs between the public choice advocates on the one hand and the ability of various élite groups to restrain or modify developments. This power struggle can best be explained by neo-élite theories with public choice prescriptions attaining recent importance. Neo-Marxists view these developments as an attack by vested interests in business and private health care companies aimed at undermining the collectivist ethos underpinning the NHS and at establishing a market in health care services, thereby increasing private profits.

The NHS may be at a crucial turning point in its evolution. The next few years will determine the extent to which élite accommodation has broken down irretrievably and the extent to which neo-Marxist explanations will prove to be dominant in accounting for events.

3 The management 'problem'

The management 'problem' in the NHS has been a persistent feature in its evolution. The quest for improved management has been the basis for a succession of reforms of the Service since its first major reorganization in 1974, and has resulted in the importation into the NHS of managerial concepts borrowed from industry and the commercial sector. (For fuller accounts of the 1974 reorganization see Haywood and Alaszewski, 1980; Hunter, 1980.) However, the major upheaval in 1974 did not signal an end to the search for improved management. Paradoxically, it fuelled yet more intensive attempts to tackle what were perceived as continuing problems in the management of health services. These led to a Royal Commission being set up in 1976, which reported in 1979. By that time, a Conservative administration had replaced Labour and had its own already partially worked-out ideas about improving the management of the Service, which gave rise to a second reorganization of the NHS in 1982 and to a battery of measures and initiatives designed to render management more efficient. These included, in addition to changes to the structure of the NHS: new machinery for reviewing health authority performance; arrangements to plan, control and monitor staffing; improvements in audit and information for both central and local monitoring; a scrutiny procedure for administrative and managerial functions; and measures to improve efficiency in specific areas such as purchasing goods and services (DHSS, 1983). These various initiatives, and others such as competitive tendering in laundry, cleaning, and catering services, culminated in October 1983 in the report from the NHS Management Inquiry team led by Roy Griffiths, Deputy Chairman and Managing Director of the Sainsbury's group.

The Griffiths report resulted in what some regard as the most profound change to take place in the NHS, namely, the introduction of general managers in place of team management. However, scarcely had this new breed of general managers settled into their posts when talk of further reform began to be heard. Sure enough, in the midst of an alleged funding crisis in the NHS in late 1987/early 1988, the Prime Minister unexpectedly announced a review of the financing and organization of the Service. This resulted in the January 1989 White Paper, *Working for*

Patients, which managed to avoid any mention of funding levels – ostensibly the reason for the review (Department of Health *et al.* 1989b). The White Paper's proposals sought to build on existing management arrangements and were intended to clarify the relationship between the central department and health authorities within a clearly defined command structure. (See Annexe.)

Why has the search for better management dominated reforms of the NHS? What particular problems are posed by the fact the NHS is a *split* organization with a bureaucratic component and a professional one? Why was a particular model of management, based essentially on private sector practice, favoured when other models, perhaps more appropriate for a human services organization, were available? We attempt to shed light on these and other questions in this chapter.

The management problem in the NHS falls into three separate, though overlapping, areas of concern: attempts to set priorities nationally which can then be made to stick locally; the distribution of resources at a micro level (macro funding issues were considered in Chapter 2); and the management approach deemed most suitable to achieving the first two. The rest of this chapter reviews developments in each of these areas. A final section assesses the utility of the four theoretical perspectives set out in Chapter 1 for interpreting events considered in this chapter.

Setting priorities

Health planning and priority setting are comparatively recent developments. While the 1962 Hospital Plan sought to establish clear procedures and guidelines for hospital building, it was not until the mid-1970s that *health* (as distinct from hospital) planning became more explicit and systematic. In 1976, the DHSS issued a consultative document on priorities for health and personal social services. It candidly acknowledged that this was 'the first time an attempt has been made to establish rational and systematic priorities throughout the health and personal social services' (DHSS, 1976, p.1). The document was principally aimed at securing an improved commitment to community care, which was generally considered to be preferable to long-stay institutional care, whether in hospital or in residential homes, for the so-called priority groups, namely the mentally ill, mentally and physically handicapped, and elderly people.

Since the 1950s, governments of all political hues have identified these care groups as meriting priority in service development and resource allocation and have enlisted the support of patient pressure groups for this position (Klein, 1983, p.81). The thrust of policy, more explicit since the mid-1970s has comprised two major emphases: first, that these care groups should be accorded priority status in relation to other areas of health and personal social services provision; and, second, that improvements in the quality of services depend on developing more balanced service systems, by which is meant an extension of services in the community (preferably home-based) and a contraction of long-stay hospital provision with its poor physical fabric, inappropriate modes of care, and record of scandals (Watkin, 1978, pp.72–83). As the 1976 priorities document stressed, and as virtually every other official statement published since has done, joint planning between health and local authorities is an essential prerequisite to a successful realization of such policy. Neither the NHS nor local government has a monopoly over community care services and collaboration between them is therefore necessary. Most of the managerial and organizational problems evident in attempts to make progress in community care have their origins in the border skirmishes between health and local authorities.

A more fundamental problem with the policy itself is evident from its mixed motives. While there was certainly a humanitarian thrust to it (the overriding wish of individuals to remain and be supported for as long as possible in their own homes), and a sense of public outrage over the conditions in many long-stay hospitals, there was also a widespread belief that community care would serve the interests of financial economy (DHSS, 1981). Analysts are divided in their views on this point. Whether community care is cheaper than institutional alternatives hinges on how the costs are calculated (for instance, are the earnings and taxes foregone by carers taken into account?) and on the quality of care provided. Nevertheless, community care is an attractive option for a government intent on reducing public spending and on rolling back the frontiers of the welfare state. Present policy is underpinned by an assumption that it is, first and foremost, the duty of the family to care for dying and dependent relatives. The family is the frontline, buttressed as and when necessary by statutory services and, increasingly, those provided by the voluntary and private sectors.

If there is disagreement about the motives of policy, there is also disagreement over whether the policy has succeeded in its aims. However, the overwhelming weight of opinion is that the policy of community care has been a failure, albeit with some notable exceptions (Working Group on Joint Planning, 1985; Audit Commission, 1986; National Audit Office, 1987; Griffiths,

1988). Even ministers acknowledge that progress has been uneven and a long haul lies ahead (Department of Health, 1989b). Of the above critiques of community care policy, the most trenchant and influential was that conducted by the Audit Commission. The Commission concluded that despite some £6 billion being spent on services for the priority groups, progress was slow and uneven across the country. Five obstacles were identified to account for this state of affairs:

- compartmentalized health and local government budgets which hampered the desired shift in resources from health to social services and did not match the requirements of community care policies;
- the absence of additional resources in the form of 'bridging' finance to meet the transitional costs involved in shifting from institutional to community care;
- the distorting effects of the Social Security funding of private residential care, which in 1988/89 was running at around £1 billion per year and still rising – perversely, this offers incentives for residential rather than domiciliary based care;
- delays, difficulties and boundary problems caused by a fragmented organizational structure; and
- the absence of staffing and training arrangements to ensure the appropriate supply of trained community based staff, and to ease the transfer of staff into the community.

Against this background, Sir Roy Griffiths in his capacity as the government's health adviser was asked at the close of 1986 to conduct a twelve month review of community care. His report, to which the government responded more than a year after its publication (see below), endorsed virtually every criticism made of community care policies and the arrangements for their implementation. A number of key recommendations were put forward:

- a clearer strategic role for central government including the appointment of a Minister for Community Care;
- a more facilitative and enabling role for social services departments as lead agencies;
- the continuing need for collaboration at local level between different agencies, including the development of case management;
- new methods of financing community care, including a specific community care grant to local authorities;
- a single gateway to publicly-financed residential care;

- greater encouragement of experiments to promote new forms of more pluralist provision;
- encouragement of joint or shared training between different professions;
- facilitation of greater consumer choice;
- clarification of the respective responsibilities of health and social care agencies; and
- the establishment of a better balance between policy aspirations and the availability of resources.

(For more detailed discussion of the Griffiths proposals and their implications for those involved in community care at all levels of government and outside government, see Hunter and Judge, 1988, Hunter, Judge and Price, 1988.)

Phillipson (1988) considers the proposals in the context of the needs of elderly people and concludes that with their emphasis on family care, they fail to acknowledge both the preferences of elderly people, who actually want formal services together with limited input from families, and the demographic changes taking place which will mean, *inter alia*, smaller, more fragmented families with fewer younger carers (mainly women in their forties) available to assume caring tasks.

The government's belated response to Sir Roy Griffiths' report came in two stages. An initial statement was presented to Parliament in July 1989 by the Secretary of State for Health. Corresponding statements were given by the Secretaries of State for Wales, Scotland and Northern Ireland. This statement was followed by a White Paper, *Caring for People*, in November 1989 which provided further details concerning the government's intentions while leaving many key questions unanswered (Department of Health *et al*, 1989a). Guidance on many of these questions and on implementation issues is being prepared by a number of task forces led by the Department of Health and Social Services Inspectorate. Outstanding questions include the crucial matter of the resources to be made available to finance community care, and the nature of the health and social care interface.

The White Paper reaffirms the government's commitment to the thrust of community care policy while conceding that progress has been unspectacular, with an inappropriate emphasis on residential care which has prevented the development of home based care. The main emphasis of the proposals is to leave unaltered the nature or responsibilities of community health services while accepting that the best way forward is to build on local authorities' existing responsibilities (see Annexe). Clearly the proposed changes amount to a major challenge for social services departments. The move to a mixed economy of provision in which local authorities will be the enablers but not necessarily always the providers of care will require a cultural revolution in the management of social services and in the way social workers conceive of their role.

Much of the above discussion of developments in community care policy in England applies more or less equally to the situation prevailing in the rest of Britain. However, in terms of implementation, there are important differences both between Scotland and Wales, and between each of them and England, which we can only summarize here; for a more detailed discussion see Gray and Hunter, 1983; Hunter and Wistow, 1987, 1988. The evidence, when the top layer of policy statements is removed, points to a substantial degree of latitude and of independent policy determination within a general but flexible framework. There are substantial divergences between England, Scotland and Wales, not simply in the pace of implementation but also, more significantly, in the fundamental goals, values and outputs associated with community care.

There are many indications that community care in Scotland lacks the resonance it enjoys elsewhere. There remains a quite distinctive service and policy profile derived from divergent professional (primarily medical) views concerning the appropriateness of long stay beds as a central component of service provision. As Martin (1984, p.66) says with regard to community care and the mentally ill in Scotland, it is 'an interesting example of quite substantial Anglo-Scottish differentiation having developed on the basis of variations in professional and administrative attitudes rather than of legislative decisions'. Despite the existence of two policy statements on health care priorities – *Scottish Health Authorities Priorities for the Eighties* (SHAPE) in 1980 and *Scottish Health Authorities Review of Priorities for the Eighties and Nineties* (SHARPEN) in 1988 – both of which stress the commitment to community care, there seems to be considerable inertia in the system, perhaps aided by Scotland's healthier resource position (see Chapter 2). Most of this extra spending has gone on hospital beds and the staff to run them. Consequently cost-push and demand-pull pressures for the development of alternatives to hospital provision have been minimized.

The approach in Wales differs considerably. The community care initiative has been pursued in two ways: first, there is an overall commitment to a community care strategy (in common with England and rather more than in Scotland); and second, there is the All Wales Strategy for the Development of Services for Mentally Handicapped People, which has no counterpart elsewhere in Britain (see Hunter and Wistow, 1987, ch. 5). The strategy is notable for its 'degree of internal coherence and political support' (Wistow, 1985, p.78). Although it is not referred to in the Griffiths agenda for community care (Griffiths, 1988), there are striking parallels between Griffiths' proposals for reform (see p.63) and the Welsh strategy.

Thus, community care services for the priority groups have been at the core of central government planning and priority setting for forty years, with a greater degree of specificity evident in the process in the mid-1970s subsequently giving way to a less explicit commitment. But there have been other national government priorities, and while these might be classed as second order priorities they merit brief mention. Indeed, an emerging paradox has been that these second order priorities have engulfed the ostensible major priority and have rendered its achievement considerably more difficult. A feature which has become particularly evident since the mid-1980s has been the large number of priorities – in the region of 47 – to which the DoH wants health authorities to respond.

The issue of priority setting is symptomatic of a more pervasive problem in the NHS. Reporting in 1979, the Royal Commission on the NHS observed:

> The absence of detailed and publicly declared principles and objectives for the NHS reflects to some degree the continuing political debate about the service. Instead of principles there are policies which change according to the priorities of the government of the day and the particular interests of the ministers concerned (1979, para. 2.5, p.9).

A decade later, the position remains virtually unchanged. Echoing many similar declarations, the Royal Commission in 1979 believed that the NHS should:

> Encourage and assist individuals to remain healthy;
> provide equality of entitlement to health services;
> provide a broad range of services of a high standard;
> provide equality of access to these services;
> provide a service free at the time of use;
> satisfy the reasonable expectations of its users;
> remain a national service responsive to local needs
> (1979, para. 2.6, p.9).

Given such a diverse and ambitious set of objectives it is little wonder that the NHS has seemed unclear of its mission. The quickening pace of technological change in medicine has only served to make the dilemma more acute. Developments in medical science have increased the range of possible interventions to prolong life or to improve its quality, but they have also served to generate increasing needs which often remain unfulfilled. Pressure is then put on politicians and managers to provide more resources for health care thereby adding further confusion to what the NHS exists to achieve. In today's health service, the inability of resources to keep pace with what can be done has sharpened the challenges in the NHS: the challenges of choosing techniques; of identifying objectives; and of establishing the efficacy of particular interventions.

Despite the persistence of the so-called priority groups described earlier, other priorities have been added to the list over the years, making it impossible to establish what precisely the real priorities are. For example, in 1984–5 health authorities were required to develop services for the priority groups but, in addition, to develop services for renal failure, coronary artery surgery, hip-joint replacement, and bone marrow transplantation. A national target of treating forty new end stage renal patients per million population by 1987 was set.

The following year – 1985/6 – the priorities remained the same. But in addition health authorities were required to develop services for drug misusers. In 1986/7, the priorities for service development remained the same as the previous year but in addition health authorities were asked to review or improve their cervical cancer screening services. The target was for all health authorities to have computerized call and recall schemes in operation and to ensure that laboratories could meet demand and avoid backlogs. Authorities were also required to develop a plan of action to combat the spread of AIDS, concentrating on high-risk groups. In 1987/8, the priorities for service development remained the same with the addition of breast cancer screening units which RHAs were to start operating by March 1988. There was also an attempt made to set specific targets, mostly in existing priority areas. For example, there was a requirement that by the end of 1988 no mentally handicapped child should need to be in a large mental handicap hospital. Health authorities were also asked to take urgent management action to reduce what were regarded as excessive waiting lists and times.

In July 1988, the DHSS issued an important circular on resource assumptions and planning guidelines, although the status of this is in some doubt following the 1989 White Paper, which has virtually nothing to say about strategy or the direction of health services. The guidelines applied to health promotion and disease prevention, acute services, services for people with a mental handicap, services for people with a mental illness, services for elderly people, services for people with physical and sensory disability, AIDS, services for drug misusers, services for alcohol misusers, maternity and prenatal services, child health services, and support services. In acute services the circular acknowledged that although they accounted for nearly half of all hospital and community health services expenditure, the Department had not issued guidance on the role of the acute sector in general. The circular proceeded to set out some guidelines, with the emphasis on health authorities planning for levels of activity in the acute sector sufficient to meet referral demand by clinically appropriate treatment.

Despite this circular, it is clear that, over the years, the list of priorities has lengthened in a somewhat directionless manner. A lengthy list of priorities is virtually useless without a weighting system or a means of ranking them. Despite mention of a corporate plan for the NHS following the Griffiths changes at the centre in 1984, nothing has come of this in England. Wales, however, has a plan and Scotland has produced a clear statement of priorities in rank order – SHARPEN (SHHD, 1988) to replace SHAPE (SHHD, 1980). However, where these documents stand in relation to the 1989 White Paper remains unclear, though potentially problematic. As Harrison, Hunter, Johnston and Wistow have pointed out:

> Principles are an essential prerequisite to service development because they give everyone involved in their development a vision coupled with a real sense of purpose and direction. The White Paper makes no mention of how its reforms will either contribute to or, as many fear, detract from the guiding principles of the NHS, while having plenty to say about specific services. There is no framework to drive the reforms, no benchmark against which to measure their success or failure, and no apparent concern with outcome or impact (1989, p.12).

In their examination of the 1989 White Paper, the Social Services Committee (1989, paras 4.59, 44.5) expressed concern over 'a growing list of priorities for the health service: too many priorities diminishes their individual importance'. The Committee called for a statement of health service priorities and their relative importance akin to the SHHD's SHARPEN report.

Because of a lack of clear political direction about ends (as distinct from means) and a steady accumulation of priorities, the NHS continues to be unsure of what its precise aims are. Are they essentially about *care*, about *cure*, about *prevention* or, as seems more likely, about some combination of all of these? Even if it is accepted in principle that the NHS should not try to do everything that is medically possible it is proving exceedingly difficult in practice to establish and keep to agreed limits. Moreover, and we return to where we began, the NHS's responsibilities in the care and health promotion sectors remain problematic. As we pointed out, implementation of the desired shift in priorities has been slow and uneven. In respect of community care, perhaps the solution lies in Griffiths' attempt in his report on community care to make a distinction between medical care and social care, with lead responsibility for social care resting with local authority social services. After considerable delay (which was believed to have its origins in the government's dislike of any solution which would strengthen the position of local authorities), the government finally announced its intentions in a statement in July 1989. It broadly accepted the Griffiths proposals in terms of giving primary responsibility for community care to local authority social services departments. As we noted above, this is broadly the direction taken in the White Paper *Caring for People*.

If progress has been negligible in regard to the priority groups, it has been virtually invisible in the promotion of good health and disease prevention. Of course, the factors which determine good health in individuals and communities are diverse and largely lie beyond the immediate influence of health professionals. However, the promotion of good health is central to the aims of the NHS as embodied in its originating Act of 1946. Moreover, the United Kingdom government is a signatory to the World Health Organization's (WHO) Health for All (HFA) by the Year 2000 initiative. The HFA initiative comprises 38 targets, many of which are aimed at promoting healthy lifestyles among populations within WHO member states. For example, target 13 states:

> By 1990, national policies in all member states should ensure that legislative, administrative and economic mechanisms provide broad intersectoral support and resources for the promotion of healthy lifestyles and ensure effective participation of the people at all levels of such policy-making (WHO, 1985, p.56).

The NHS ostensibly has an important contribution to make to the achievement of HFA. Yet, as the Royal Commission on the NHS pointed out, and as *Working for Patients* seems to endorse, the NHS has always been primarily a treatment service. Repeated calls to shift the emphasis have met with little response in terms of an identifiable change in priorities. Moreover, where a wider definition of health does appear, the *individualism* of modern health problems is stressed. Policy is based on attempts to change individual behaviour (Research Unit in Health and Behavioural Change, 1989); such pronouncements often have a merely symbolic appeal, with negligible impact on the direction of policy. For instance, simply advocating that more intersectoral coordination is desirable will not by itself make it happen. There is a tension, too, in the emphasis on individualism of those on the political right, which perceives health problems as the responsibility of individuals and their lifestyles, and the view of the political left which stresses the structural determinants of ill-health, which require attention to social and economic reforms in order to change the environment which negatively impinges on public health. (Norway in the mid-1970s provided an example of innovation in the formulation of a national nutrition and food policy inspired by a structuralist perspective (Ziglio, 1986). The intention to allow diet and health considerations to influence the production, supply and pricing of food is novel and remains unique in Western developed countries. A structuralist perspective also underpins the WHO's HFA strategy.) The 1989 White Paper proposals rest firmly on the individualistic perspective.

While *care* has struggled, largely unsuccessfully, for supremacy over *cure* in the NHS, issues relating to health itself as distinct from health care and services have received even less attention. During the lifetime of the NHS there have been significant improvements in the health of the population. But it is important to remember that the NHS has been a modest contributor to these compared with the efforts in other sectors of public policy (McKeown, 1980). Support for the NHS as an institution can all too easily lead to an inflated assessment of its impact on health status.

The government's plan for primary health care which appeared in a White Paper, *Promoting Better Health*, in late 1988 were designed, *inter alia*, to promote health and prevent illness. The foreword to the White Paper emphasizes the need to 'shift the emphasis in primary care from the treatment of illness to the promotion of health and the prevention of disease' (DHSS *et al*, 1987). However, as Marks (1988) has pointed out, the subsequent imposition of charges for eye tests and dental examinations is at variance with this aim. For general medical services, a number of incentives are proposed to encourage preventive activities. GPs will be offered incentives to meet preventive targets as well as fees for holding health promotion clinics. They will be required to provide basic screening services for their practice populations, and encouraged to provide comprehensive regular care for elderly people.

While the preventive emphasis of the White Paper has been generally welcomed, concern has been expressed over some aspects of the approach. For example, the *Lancet* (1987) noted:

> Many of the preventative activities proposed are of unproven effectiveness, and direct attention from the more difficult and basic issues of acceptable standards of service provision and diagnostic and treatment skills (p. 1308).

Noting the White Paper's welcome emphasis on the need to improve the accountability of independent contractors working in primary health care, Marks (1988) is critical of the gaps in, and narrow focus of, the proposals:

> By narrowing the focus of health promotion into the role of individuals and their GPs and by narrowing the focus of general practice into preventative care, some complex policy debates are neatly evaded (p.17).

Among the debates overlooked is the provision of appropriate care for the priority groups discussed earlier, and the place of primary care as the key component in WHO's HFA strategy.

The government sees its 1989 White Paper proposals for the Family Practitioner Services (see Annexe) as building on the earlier White Paper.

It has been suggested that changes in health policy in the coming decades are likely to be determined either by a continuing adherence to cost-containment, with the emphasis on savings and cuts in spending dressed up as improvements in efficiency, or by the emergence of a new health policy agenda aimed at promoting health. The first more of the same scenario has the virtue of consistency and of being more readily implementable especially if the vested interests opposed to such a strategy – principally the medical profession but also other producer groups – are turned in line with the management changes which have occurred over the past seven or eight years and those proposed in *Working for Patients*. The second scenario 'implies a need for a shift in health priorities and resource allocation not just confined to the health sector: a task far from being a straightforward one in most Western developed countries' (Research Unit in Health and Behavioural Change, 1989, p.143). Within the NHS it implies the pursuit of an appropriate mix of the various activities considered earlier in this section: curing, caring, prevention and health promotion. In arriving at such a mix, policymakers would be required to come to terms with the internal and external conflicts that any reallocation of resources and shift in priorities generates for professional power and organizational control.

The distribution of resources

The issue of funding health services was the subject of the last chapter. It is necessary, however, to consider separately the *distribution* of resources. The problem of distributing resources within the NHS is an issue as old as the Service itself. The desire to achieve a more equitable distribution of resources is a basic tenet of the NHS model. Its architect Aneurin Bevan wrote in 1945: 'We have got to achieve as nearly as possible a uniform standard of service for all.' In Bevan's view, only through a *national* service in which resources were allocated according to centrally determined criteria could the state ensure that 'an equally good service is available everywhere'.

Despite the goal of uniformity across the country, until 1976 the basic expenditure patterns remained as they had been in the days before the NHS existed. Even today, large geographical variations in the provision of health care – in particular the hospital service – remain at all levels, region, district and unit; they have been inherited from the pre-NHS era. As Buxton and Klein (1978, p.2) argued in a report prepared for the Royal Commission on the NHS: 'The magnitudes of these differences become amplified as one considers smaller territorial units.'

The persistence of geographical inequalities in resource distribution reflects a mix of policy inertia ('to him who hath shall more be given') and demographic drag (that is, the failure to adapt resource allocation to population changes), to use Buxton and Klein's terms. The policy of the central health departments was for many years an incremental approach to budgeting which perpetuated the status quo; the yearly growth additions to RHA allocations were largely based on existing commitments, with the inevitable result of perpetuating inherited inequalities. The division of the budget could have been characterized as last year's allocation plus an allowance for growth, plus an allowance for political pressures. The dynamics of the process have been well captured by the notion referred to in Chapter 1 as incremental politics.

The demographic drag factor was particularly important at subregional level; by this is meant the failure to adapt the allocation of revenue and capital funds to population changes and movements. The worst cases of relative over-provision are to be found in inner city areas where sharp falls in population levels have not been accompanied by a shrinkage in, or rationalization of, health facilities. Further examples are those areas which have attracted large numbers of elderly people who make additional demands on health care services but for whom no allowance is made in the allocation of resources.

It was not until the late 1960s that policymakers put inequality in the regional distribution of resources at the top of their agenda. The first such resource allocation formula, the hospital revenue allocation formula, was introduced in 1970. According to this, hospital revenue was allocated on a basis of three regional indicators: bed stock, case flow and population.

Some years later, in 1975, a more thoroughgoing attempt to redress regional imbalances was introduced. A resource allocation working party (RAWP) was set up by the government to establish 'a method of securing . . . a pattern of distribution responsive objectively, equitably and efficiently . . . to relative need'. RAWP produced its interim formula in 1975 and a revised version in 1976 (Resource Allocation Working Party, 1976). It formed the basis on which resources were allocated to RHAs in England from 1976 to 1989. Separate formulae apply in Wales, Scotland and Northern Ireland but they all share the same policy objective, namely to equalize resource allocation across territories so as to ensure equal access to services for those in equal need. All four formulae have adopted the same broad principle, that resource allocation should be based on population size, weighted to reflect the need for services. They differ in their methods of weighting of the population and in the services included in the formula allocations. The RAWP formula is based on seven criteria by which the relative need for health care could be established:

- population size;
- age and sex structure of the population;
- mortality (as a proxy for morbidity, or illness) of the population;
- cost of providing care;
- cross boundary flow of patients between health authorities;
- cost of medical and dental education; and
- distribution of buildings, plant and equipment.

Except insofar as already reflected by mortality, the formula does not reflect the effect of social deprivation on the need for hospital and community services. It has been criticized for this on the grounds that factors such as poor housing, unemployment and poverty have a greater effect on health than other conventional measures included in the formula.

The innovative feature of the formulae was the attempt to measure the relative needs of regional populations for health service resources and to ignore historical legacies. Not surprisingly, given the complexity and ambitious nature of the task, the formulae have not escaped criticism, both at the level of the assumptions underpinning them and at the level of their technical construction. Implementation of the formulae has been based on incremental growth rates determined by each region's distance above or below its target allocation. The speed at which regions have moved towards their targets is referred to as the 'pace of change'. Generally this pace has been gradual; the targets may have represented quite a major redistribution, but they have been approached incrementally. Pace depends ultimately on political will and commitment. Until recently a broad consensus has existed across political parties concerning the importance and necessity of a redistribution of resources from the better-off regions to the poor ones, but a persistent difficulty from the start has been achieving such an aim at a time of general resource constraints in the NHS.

In the last two to three years, there has been mounting criticism of the RAWP formula. The two principal criticisms are, firstly that equalizing resource distribution does not necessarily mean an equalization of the provision and availability of health care, and secondly that the formulae do not apply at the sub-regional level where inequalities are often much greater in magnitude. The government, as part of its package of reforms for the NHS announced in *Working for Patients* has decided to heed some of these criticisms and to replace the RAWP formula in 1990 with a system based on each region's resident population, arguing that eleven of the fourteen RHAs are within 3 per cent of their RAWP targets and therefore that the major differences have gone.

At sub-regional level also, a new system is seen as necessary. In future, both regions and districts are to be funded on per head of population basis weighted to reflect the health and age distribution of the population including the number of elderly people and the relative cost of providing services. The four Thames Regions will receive a higher level of funding – up to 3 per cent higher per head of population – to reflect the higher costs of and demands on services in London. It can be argued that such a move represents a victory for the London area which was the most over-provided and therefore suffered under RAWP. The effect of the new funding system will be to reverse the impact of the RAWP formula by channelling resources to areas of growing population such as the South East, South West, East Anglia and North Yorkshire. Areas of falling population are likely to experience problems in maintaining and developing services.

The new arrangements have been introduced in order to facilitate the creation of a provider market in health care whereby regions and districts will be able to purchase services directly from each other (see Annexe). The proposals derive from Enthoven's (1985) notion of an internal market, intended to stimulate competition between hospital services and GP services as a way of increasing efficiency by providing incentives to doctors. Internal markets entail a sharper recognition of responsibilities and costs which, in turn, demands particular management skills. This leads us to consider one of the enduring concerns in the history of the NHS, namely the quest for improved management.

Managing the NHS: selected highlights

It is not the purpose of this review to supply a comprehensive history of health service management. Detailed accounts of these developments may be found elsewhere (Allsop, 1984, ch.4; Harrison, 1988a, ch.2; Levitt and Wall, 1984), and we make some reference in Chapter 4 to the *impact* of the more recent changes. But some mapping of the terrain is desirable in order to make clear the nature of the landscape being surveyed. The developments that have occurred in management are broadly similar across the United Kingdom, notwithstanding differences in the timing and in nuances of the reforms in each of the four countries comprising the United Kingdom (see Annexe).

As noted above, interest in improved management began to gather momentum in the late 1960s and early 1970s. In part, it reflected a more general concern evident at the time across the public sector particularly in central and local government. An essentially managerial ideology of reform permeated the public sector as a whole throughout this period. Heclo and Wildavsky (1981), in their account of Whitehall, refer to the period as the New Rationalism. It reflected mounting concern with the alleged poor performance of the government machine. The Conservative administration at the time believed that government and big business were not so different and that government therefore required a modern management ethos in order to thrive. Echoes of this belief were to reverberate repeatedly throughout the NHS from the early 1970s to the present. Indeed, to appreciate recent events in the NHS and to put them in their proper context it is necessary to give a sketch of earlier changes in its management (see Annexe for a description of the present NHS structure).

It is no easy task explaining why the quest for improved management and the adoption of a particular management style captured the hearts and minds of so many. The antecedents are multiple and complex (Pollitt, 1990). What is clear is that the managerial ethos was not the product of any systematic empirical study of the NHS, and that occupational politics was an important factor (Harrison, 1988a, pp.27–8).

The 1960s and 1970s were characterized by a general belief in the efficacy of organization structure and management training as a means of producing better management in the public sector; better management career structures were seen as the answer to the problem, almost irrespective of what the problem was. Indeed, in the extreme case the absence of managerial careers was seen *as* the problem; the Salmon Report took it as axiomatic that nurses' status was too low, and all its proposals flowed from this (Ministry of Health and Scottish Home and Health Department 1966, p.7). Increasing managerial specialization was another manifestation of the same assumption, as was the increased attention paid to training and education of managers (see, for instance, King's Fund Working Party, 1977).

Claims for managerial roles and equality of status with administrators therefore became the strategy by which the health professions other than medicine sought to advance themselves;

> Each professional group – which was of course heavily represented on the working party concerned with its particular specialty – was naturally ready to welcome a form of organisation which provided more numerous and more lucrative opportunities of promotion for its members (Watkin, 1975, p.349).

There was another point of view. An important, though not widely known, report was published in Scotland in 1966 which addressed the need to improve the administrative practice of hospital boards (Scottish Health Services Council, 1966); much of the managerial philosophy and quest for greater efficiency and effectiveness which emerged in 1984 when the Griffiths management reforms were introduced, may be found in this report. The Farquharson-Lang report, after the name of the committee's chairman, called for increased standards of management ability from officers and a clearer distinction between their functions and those of board (health authority) members. A report from a joint working party of the Institute of Hospital Administrators and the

King's Fund made similar recommendations (Joint Working Party, 1967). Pre-dating the introduction of general management by twenty years or so, Farquharson-Lang's most controversial recommendation was for the establishment of a chief executive post in place of the administrator to be filled by either a professional or medically qualified administrator. Such an individual would be in charge of all professional personnel – a position of command which had no parallel in the NHS at that time as far as medical staff were concerned, since each consultant enjoyed virtual autonomy. But the constituency for such heretical thoughts was weak both in Scotland and England and nothing came of the report's proposals. On the contrary, events moved in the opposite direction.

Between 1974 and 1984 consensus management teams comprising an administrator, a treasurer, one or more doctors and a nurse operated in the NHS. Prior to 1974, chief officers meeting as a group had no formal authority, and decisions which required formal authority greater than that possessed by an individual officer had to be taken to the health authority. The development of teams in part formalized what was already happening in health authorities informally in the pre-1974 structure, so that under consensus management the management group was vested with a collective authority to take decisions and enjoyed a corporate existence and responsibility.

The consensus management group concept enhanced the status of the nurse and treasurer in health service management. They were equal members of the group alongside the doctor and the administrator. Indeed, one of the major objections to the introduction of general management a decade later was that it put at risk the management gains achieved by nurses. The 1974 management reforms resulted in quite substantial adjustments occurring in the respective responsibilities of officers and health authority members, the upshot of which was that a great deal of decisionmaking lay not with authority members but with officers.

The responsibility was on consensus management groups of officers not to present a case to the health authority in their individual capacities, as happened prior to 1974, but to agree the right decision among themselves first. In short, health authorities were supposed to be concerned with principles and their officers gave effect to these through a wide range of delegated and detailed decisions. Therefore, not only did the 1974 changes seek to improve management in the health service, but a chief means of achieving such an improvement was to realign the responsibilities of lay members with those of professional officers so that the latter exercised greater scope over the business of the health authority. The effect of all the changes at this time was that the role of authority members contracted considerably while that of officers greatly expanded. In practice, in Brown's terms (1975, p.203), lay members were 'restricted to a *policy approving and monitoring role*, leaving *detailed management and the formulation of policy* to officers' (italics added).

The 1974 reorganization of the NHS gave rise to considerable criticism, particularly in England. Three areas were the focus of the critics' attention: first, emphasis on a particular model of 'scientific management', derived from sections of industry which was viewed as inappropriate to human services like health; second, the uncertain and confused role of health authority members – were they managers, or representatives of the community, or both?; and third, problems arising from the consensus approach to management and decisionmaking.

Consensus management was viewed with considerable scepticism by those concerned by the lack of a unified authority in the NHS and the length of time taken to reach decisions (for a review see Harrison, 1982). It was perceived to be at the root of what many observers regarded as the fundamental flaw in the 1974 model, namely, the absence of clear responsibility: there was nowhere for the buck to stop (Maynard, 1983, p.36). This criticism formed the thrust of Griffiths' argument some ten years later when he wrote that the NHS existed in a state of 'institutionalised stagnation' (NHS Management Inquiry, 1983). It led directly to the recommendation for general managers to be appointed at all levels of the Service. It has been argued by Klein among others (1974a) that the creation of consensus management teams was the only way out of the *impasse* resulting from professional intransigence over the desirability of a chief executive figure who would run the Service within each authority in much the same way as local authority chief executives managed services in their localities. As Farquharson-Lang discovered some years earlier, a major difficulty over having chief executives in the NHS has been the inability to agree on who should be eligible for such posts.

Apart from those who believed that consensus management had led to weak management, sapping individual responsibility, there were those who argued that the management changes introduced in 1974 went too far in terms of importing inappropriate management concepts. Burns (1981), for instance, was critical of the 'recrudescence of hard line managerialism: and primitive, already outdated managerialism at that'. He contrasted the supporting, enabling role of management with the controlling hierarchical one and feared that the latter had been in the ascendant since 1974. Draper and Smart (1974) were of the opinion that structures of the type underpinning the 1974 model of management would become rule bound, inflexible and insensitive to the needs of, and changes in, the world around them. They argued that management change had done little to affect the real quality of health care for any group of the population. What was needed, they suggested, was an alteration in the pattern of social relations associated with the process of medical care. Such changes might occur more readily if the public had the opportunity to participate in preventing or alleviating health problems.

Moreover, the rumblings from service practitioners, who were critical of what they regarded as an unnecessarily cumbersome and overbearing structure, became sufficiently loud for a Royal Commission to be set up in 1976 only two years after the NHS had been reorganized. (Other factors also contributed: increasing trade union activity and a dispute over the place of private practice in the NHS.) The Commission's remit was to look at the management of the financial and manpower resources of the NHS. It reported in 1979, by which time the Labour government had been replaced by a Conservative administration which largely ignored the five hundred page tome. A consultative document, *Patients First* (DHSS and Welsh Office, 1979) set out ministers' thoughts. Hard on the heels of the English document came versions for Scotland and Northern Ireland; Wales objected to its perfunctory treatment in two paragraphs in the 1979 document and a separate Welsh version was issued (Welsh Office, 1980).

Patients First advocated simplification of the structure of the NHS but did not put forward any proposals for reforming its management. Indeed, ministers were emphatic that consensus management teams were to stay. They were, however, anxious to improve the performance of teams by stressing the responsibility of individual managers. The thrust of *Patients First* was to allow local health authorities greater discretion over the services for which they were responsible in order to meet the particular needs of their communities. At the same time, central government was to withdraw from detailed intervention in the affairs of health authorities and exercise a self-denying ordinance. There was to be delegation to unit level and, to simplify arrangements, a tier of organization was abolished from April 1982.

Even before this reorganization was complete it was becoming increasingly difficult for ministers to maintain this hands-off stance. Reports from the influential and respected House of Commons Public Accounts Committee, and the Social Services Committee, coupled with pressure from the Treasury, the Prime

Minister and the Confederation of British Industry, all focused political attention on the lack of clear accountability in the NHS (CBI, 1981; Harrison, 1988a, pp.91–9; Hunter, 1983c). There was a feeling that at a time of acute economic depression and of growing resource restraints the NHS must do its bit and demonstrate that it was using existing resources efficiently and to maximum effect, and that national policy priorities were being implemented. Also, an informal 1979 agreement between ministers to the effect that the NHS should be preserved from reductions in real resources ran out in 1981–2. It was, therefore, not politically tenable for the DHSS to be advocating a hands-off policy at such a time.

Despite the introduction of such measures as efficiency savings, Rayner Scrutinies, and Performance Indicators (Harrison ,1988a, pp.56–9), mounting concerns and criticisms led to an internal management inquiry. The original intention had been to undertake a review of 'manpower' but this was not acceptable to Roy Griffiths. Former permanent secretary at the DHSS, Sir Kenneth Stowe, has noted 'the seemingly endless expansion in the size of the hospital workforce, which was bound to make it that much harder to constrain public expenditure' (Stowe, 1989, p.51). The NHS industrial dispute of 1982 had involved a strike in hospitals and led the government to conclude that an inquiry into NHS staffing was needed. In Stowe's words, 'the seeds were sown' which produced the Griffiths management inquiry. It is not clear why the government accepted an inquiry agenda reshaped by Griffiths. There are two possible explanations: first, it took a considerable time to find somebody suitable to lead the inquiry – had Roy Griffiths refused, the DHSS would have had to start its search again; second, by instituting a review, the secretary of state could keep at bay critics of the Department's policy and assure them that the government took seriously the criticisms coming from the Treasury, Parliament and elsewhere. The inquiry team was set up in February 1983 under the leadership of Roy Griffiths. In October of that year, he submitted a twenty-three page letter to the then Secretary of State for Social Services, Norman Fowler (NHS Management Inquiry, 1983). It was extensively leaked, which left the government with little alternative but to publish the document. It was a report intended for action rather than for lengthy consultation or deliberation. The contrast with the long report by the Royal Commission on the NHS could not have been more striking. Despite opposition from the BMA and Royal College of Nursing (RCN), though with IHSM support (Social Services Committee, 1984), ministers promptly agreed to its major recommendations with the result that in under a year steps were taken to introduce the proposals in the NHS (see p.166).

The Griffiths report combined diagnosis with prescription. Its thrust was that the NHS suffered from institutionalized stagnation, the result of a labyrinthine consultation process and a system of consensus management teams which gave the right of veto to each team member. Griffiths' charge that the Service lacked a clearly-defined general management function caught the spirit of the times. Even so – and often overlooked – Griffiths did not seek to diminish the value of consensus among managers (as distinct from formalized consensus decisionmaking); a general manager was to 'harness the best of the consensus management approach and avoid the worst of the problems it can present'. However, it was not spelt out what precisely this meant in practice and in the implementation of the proposal the notion of consensus was little heard. Nor was it much in evidence as the organizational structures and management arrangements were put in place around the country. A puzzle to be solved is what, if anything, had changed between 1979, when the government had rejected the proposition that each health authority should appoint a chief executive on the grounds that such an appointment 'would not be compatible with the professional independence required' (DHSS and Welsh Office, 1979), and 1983, when the secretary of state moved promptly to implement Griffiths' proposal for general managers at all levels of the NHS? We return to this question below.

Griffiths' recommendations were directed at the health departments as well as the NHS itself. The report expressed concern over the way in which the centre became involved in the detailed affairs of the Service. There was both too much and too little intervention; the Service suffered from too many fussy directives on operational matters and too little clear direction on overall strategy. These observations echoed those set out in an earlier review of RHA/DHSS relationships completed by three RHA chairmen at the invitation of the then minister of state, Dr David Owen (Regional Chairmen, 1976). Griffiths proposed a Supervisory Board which would set the strategy for the NHS and a Management Board which would give effect to the strategy. The Management Board was designed to keep the DHSS at arm's length from the Service and prevent or minimize interference by civil servants and ministers. However, and following an internal struggle for control of the Board, since it was itself located *within* the Department, many observers doubted its ability to operate with the necessary degree of independence. Even its former chief executive, seconded from IBM, Len Peach, acknowledged that the management of the NHS could not be divorced from politics

(Peach, 1988). The first chairman of the Management Board, Victor Paige, was uncomfortable operating in such a context and resigned. The 1989 White Paper virtually endorses the unanimous conclusion reached by outside observers that the Management Board had failed. In their place are a Management Executive with a new chief executive drawn from the NHS, and a Policy Board. Whether the changes (which replicate the original Griffiths proposals) will lead to ministers standing back from detailed interference remains to be seen. Former DHSS permanent secretary, Sir Kenneth Stowe, is unequivocal in his view that the chief executive will find life no different from Victor Paige (Stowe, 1989):

> Government never was and never will be like commercial business. The process of trying to bring some of the virtues of the business approach into central functions . . . was, and will continue to be, demanding and fretful (p.54).

Griffiths also had a great deal to say about the role of clinicians in management and budgeting. The intention was to make doctors more aware of the costs they incurred each time they decided upon a course of treatment. To this end, doctors were to be encouraged to participate closely in the preparation and holding of 'management budgets' and to employ information resulting from these to improve their use of resources. The ideas about management budgeting were expressed in the Griffiths report in fairly general terms; they involved allocating resources (i.e. budgets) to consultants and gave them specific responsibility for managing programmes of clinical care. Unlike some earlier experiments, the schemes made clinicians responsible for indirect as well as direct costs and did not always allow budget-holders to employ underspendings for their own purposes (virement) (Pollitt *et al*, 1988, pp.215–19).

For management budgeting to succeed a number of prerequisites had to be satisfied. First, there had to be a willingness among clinicians to cooperate in the development of the systems to generate the relevant data. A further prerequisite was a genuine commitment from the health authority, general manager and other senior managers to see management budgeting developed. Early experiments in four sites were not spectacularly successful. Problems were also encountered in a larger number of 'second generation' pilot sites, and the scheme was relaunched in 1986 under the new rubric of 'resource management', with greater emphasis on the human behavioural dimension of change and on clinical as well as financial information (Pollitt *et al*, 1988).

Commenting on Griffiths' prescription for change in the NHS, one general manager asserted: 'Griffiths wants to change the culture. He is trying to do a very much bigger task than just appointing a general manager' (Social Services Committee, 1984, p.72). The general manager would be personally accountable for securing action, a major change for health service managers. Professional chief officers would continue to be directly accountable to the health authority, and have a right of access to it, but only on the provision and quality of professional advice. On other matters, they would be accountable to the general manager for the day-to-day performance of their management functions. A former DHSS permanent secretary, Sir Patrick Nairne, has argued that the Griffiths report marked a 'shift from structural reorganization to managerial reform' (Nairne, 1983, p.243). Part of this shift reflected, in his view, a government intent upon increasing managerial efficiency rather than altering the structural arrangements. But is this an adequate explanation of a fundamental shift in government thinking which had hitherto shown no signs of overthrowing consensus management or is it a convenient and tidy *post hoc* rationalization of events?

It is time to return to the question we posed earlier: why did the government pounce with such enthusiasm upon general management, when less than four years earlier the same government, albeit under a different secretary of state, had rejected chief executives and any shift from consensus management on the grounds that this would displease the (principally medical) professionals? There is no simple answer to this puzzling question. Even if one accepts Nairne's explanation that the government shifted from tinkering with the structure of the NHS to a commitment to making that structure work more effectively, one is still left with the question of why such a change took place. A possible explanation lies in the criticism that the DHSS lacked sufficient grip on the NHS and that health authorities were insufficiently accountable to ministers. In addition, the Treasury was raising questions about the growing NHS budget at a time when one of the government's highest priorities was to contain and reduce levels of public spending. If the NHS was to be treated as a deserving case for additional funds, then it had to demonstrate that it was using its existing allocation to best effect. Improved management was the secretary of state's weapon to demonstrate to the Treasury that the DHSS took its obligations seriously. In all this, the professions were effectively overlooked at a national consultative level. From a position adopted back in 1948 where their sensibilities and freedoms were not to be disturbed, the government no longer regarded this implicit understanding with the professions as sacrosanct, particularly when it was intent upon decisive action to stave off further interference by the Treasury in the DHSS's affairs.

It is not clear whether the government had already made up its mind that general management was the answer or whether it simply seized upon Griffiths' prescription because of its instant appeal and timeliness in terms of the negotiations with the Treasury. Possibly, like the elephant, the DHSS only knew what it wanted when it saw it. This is perhaps a more plausible explanation particularly since, as we noted earlier, Griffiths was initially approached to carry out a staffing review. He refused on the grounds that staffing problems were symptomatic of management failure (Harrison, 1988a, p.103). Griffiths therefore shifted the reform agenda although the government was seemingly easily persuaded that a management review was what was really needed.

All this rather suggests that Nairne's tidy explanation is perhaps best relegated to the realms of *post hoc* rationalization. If there was broad agreement that the management problem in the NHS had still to be resolved, there was less certainty over how this might be done. The final solution awaited the outcome of the Griffiths inquiry.

In the management changes that have occurred since 1983, it is important to distinguish between form and substance. The changes have been long on form but rather shorter on substance. While formal changes need to be documented and the reasons for them understood, it is necessary to go behind the facade to consider their impact on the power relationships which are a key feature of any organization. For instance, the Griffiths reforms were explicitly directed towards improving performance, offering greater consumer responsiveness, ensuring more effective implementation of plans and priorities, and securing improved resource use. Crisper management was to be the means to these ends. However, achieving them meant confronting and modifying the interests and influence of various groups of actors, notably clinicians.

Some five years on, it is too early to pass final judgement on the Griffiths reforms although work in hand suggests that their impact upon the medical arena remains weak (Harrison, Hunter, Marnoch and Pollitt, 1989a, 1989b). This interim finding, and the cumulative research evidence from numerous interventions to improve NHS management over the years, suggest that it is not possible to isolate the reality of management practices from the context in which they operate. In particular, the shift from consensus management to general management demands more than simply a relabelling exercise, or changes in health services which leave the substantive core (clinical) activity undisturbed. Indeed, in seeking to control the medicine–management interface in order to modify medical practice, the 1989 White Paper acknowledges that the management changes to date do not go far enough. The proposals are aimed at addressing this unfinished business and at ensuring that doctors are held accountable for their actions in a way not countenanced in previous NHS reforms (see Chapter 4 and Annexe). As Harrison (1988a, p.122) concludes from his review of changes in managing the NHS up to the 1989 White Paper, while NHS managers are now more clearly agents of government than prior to the Griffiths reforms and although 'the frontier of control between government and doctors has shifted a little, in favour of the former, there is as yet little evidence that managers have secured greater control over doctors'. Much of the impetus behind the 1989 White Paper proposals can be seen as an attempt to secure such a shift. Hardly surprising, therefore, that the health care professions led by the British Medical Association are virtually unanimous in their opposition to such proposals. We shall return to the basis of medical influence in Chaper 4.

Before leaving the management changes which have been introduced at various times since 1974, it is necessary to comment on those themes which have run through all the changes: the tension between efficiency and control, the attempts between 1979 and 1981 (and again in 1989 with the White Paper proposals) to advocate decentralization as a way of partially 'depoliticizing' the seemingly intractable problem of managing the NHS in a situation where demands appear forever to outstrip available resources, and the moves since 1979 to regard the problems in the NHS not as funding problems but as management problems. By focusing on the latter, blame can be diffused, to paraphrase Klein (1983, p.140), since if the problem is perceived as a management one then it becomes the responsibility of the NHS and not of ministers.

A recurring theme throughout all these changes in NHS management has been the desire for improved efficiency in the use of resources and in the provision of health care services. A DHSS report, *Health Care and its Costs* (DHSS, 1983), expresses the issue well. With growing pressures from, *inter alia*, an ageing population for more health care:

> It is important that the health service should use the resources available to it as efficiently as possible in order to get the best value out of the increased finances made available and to develop at the fastest practicable rate (Preface).

To secure improvements in efficiency, the government's recent policy has comprised a battery of centre-driven, top-down initiatives and controls, including a regional review system, performance indicators, policy scrutinies, cost improvement programmes, competitive tendering, and changes in management structures and processes (Harrison, 1988a, ch.4). There is an underlying assumption that these controls will generate improved efficiency throughout the NHS at all levels. The evidence, some of which we have reviewed, is somewhat equivocal on the matter but leaves the observer in no doubt that the reforms have been found wanting in many respects. But the problem is not of recent origin and lies at the heart of centre–periphery relations in the NHS (Hunter, 1983c). The health policy arena is marked by oscillations over time between firm central control at one extreme and permissive local discretion at the other. The desire for control may emanate from the health departments, the RHA, the DHA, or may occur at the periphery in terms of a general manager's attempt to influence or modify the behaviour of clinicians.

It is in relation to centre–periphery relations that the problem of control on the one hand and devolution on the other is most apparent. The centre lacks adequate control over the periphery's performance, but at the same time is quite incapable of managing such a complex undertaking as the NHS, although it is rarely prepared publicly to acknowledge this fact. Decentralization therefore has its attractions for a minister anxious to push problems away from the ministerial desk and be freed from the constant glare of bad publicity. As we noted earlier, between 1979 and 1982, and following a long interventionist phase between 1962 and 1979, an attempt was made to devolve responsibility to local health authorities. A philosophy of *laissez-faire* began to replace the faith in planning and in direct intervention by the centre in local affairs. Klein (1981) suggested that the 1979 reforms made 'a virtue of necessity – i.e. acknowledging central government's difficulties in trying to control the periphery'. But the new philosophy of devolution created a vacuum in the chain of accountability – a feature not lost on the Treasury, the Public Accounts Committee and the Social Services Committee, all of whom moved quickly to criticize the hands-off stance, and in the end, to vitiate it. The 1989 White Paper refers to the need to decentralize responsibility as far as possible and seeks to achieve this by introducing market principles into the NHS, yet is also emphatic about the need for a clear chain of command from the top to the bottom of the NHS. The combination of these notions may represent a sophisticated attempt to find a solution to a problem which has dogged the NHS from its inception.

However, we have severe doubts about the extent to which a devolved system of health care is possible, whatever its intrinsic appeal to ministers anxious to reduce the high political profile which the NHS has acquired. The dilemma is that as long as the NHS remains centrally funded, there must be limits on how far the centre can realistically relax controls. As we have seen, MPs, not to mention the Treasury, would not have in any other way:

> [The secretary of state] will manage the service – with only a vague idea of what the words 'manage' and 'service' mean – and, by implication, be responsible for making good any deficiency. For so long as Exchequer funding remains the main or only source of money, that expectation will remain. But it cannot be 'managed' in any meaningful sense of the term at this level (Stowe, 1989, p.70).

A final theme for comment is the tendency to regard problems in the NHS as managerial in origin rather than as financial. The NHS is not unique in being perceived in these terms: all public sector services have in recent years been subject to the same presumption (Pollitt, 1990). The government's philosophy follows the lines of the new right theories outlined in Chapter 1: services have grown bloated and there is considerable scope for reassessing the uses to which resources are put. In the absence of effective outcome measures, it is difficult to challenge such a view although many, notably the Social Services Committee, have tried. By structuring the debate in narrow, technical managerial terms the government has sought to deflect attention from more overtly political concerns about funding levels. Thus the 1989 White Paper asserts that the NHS is well funded and that the challenge is to utilize available resources more intensively and efficiently; any additional resources will have to come from individuals purchasing their own care.

The NHS management problem, then, comprises a number of elements: achieving a balance between centralization and decentralization; trying to shift attention from a problem perceived as under-funding to one perceived as under-management; and, in particular, the need to control the freedom enjoyed by clinicians to incur expenditure.

At this point it is appropriate to pause in order to assess the utility of our four theories in interpreting the events described in this chapter: shifting priorities in health care, resource distribution at local level, and the search for better management.

Managing the NHS: an interpretation

None of our chosen theories fully accounts for the various developments in management that have taken place in the NHS, although each sheds some light on these. Before we consider our four theories, however, it is necessary to mention briefly a type of theory which we have not dealt with elsewhere: rational theory. We mention this here because rational theory is ubiquitous in managers' own language; it contains a unitary view of organizational relationships within the Service. Tensions, or clashes of interests, are perceived as irrational and are defined as technical problems: for example, as failure in communication, poor information, cognitive failure and so on. Indeed, if the early developments in management budgeting are examined, including the reasons accounting for their failure, these factors are uppermost (Ham and Hunter, 1988; Pollitt et al, 1988). Although such theories of rationality are somewhat discredited in academic circles (Patten and Pollitt, 1980), the ideas live on in much current management practice and among the kind of businessmen and management consultants who advise governments. Classical management theory still informs much of the language employed by reformers and, as we saw above, the present structure of the NHS is largely justified in terms of it.

The shift in priorities from institutional care to community care for vulnerable groups reflects the ascendancy of certain views within policy networks involving professionals and, more specifically professional advisers, within the health departments, as well as certain consumer pressure groups. To this extent, neo-pluralists can account for why innovative concepts such as normalization and ordinary life concepts in respect of mentally handicapped people have found their way onto policy agendas and into numerous policy statements. But the fact that their implementation has been uneven and that governments have not sought to implement them vigorously may have more to do with neo-élitist explanations which confirm the dominance of institutional agendas by particular entrenched interests. In the NHS, acute sector interests have successfully resisted any challenge from competing sectors and have protected budgets from being reallocated to different priorities, despite some local successes in implementing the shift in priorities. We also noted the differences in this area between the constituent parts of the United Kingdom, which we argued were substantially due to élite administrative and professional attitudes rather than to government views.

In regard to health promotion and the move to implement the WHO's Health for All strategy, the neo-pluralist approach has something to offer. As we suggested, successful health promotion policies go far beyond the NHS or health care sector and demand changes in many other policy sectors which touch on a large variety of social and economic interests. Not the least affected is big business and its attempt to prevent, not necessarily overtly, health promotion policies (which extend, incidentally, into such areas as food production) being seen as threatening to its interests. Such observations can also, of course, be interpreted by neo-Marxists, for whom the relegation of health promotion and the HFA strategy to the category of symbolic policymaking is entirely predictable and not at all surprising. Within a capitalist system there are strict limits in terms of how far governments will confront business interests if these are likely to have a damaging effect on trading and profits.

At first sight, public choice theories are also useful. Since hospital services form the bulk of NHS provision, it would be expected that welfare-maximizing bureaucrats would seek to defend and expand them rather than favouring non-institutional activities such as health promotion. Similarly, hospital care would be favoured rather than community care. But those theories do not shed light on such topics as intra-United Kingdom policy variation.

Turning to our second topic for this chapter, resource allocation, it is immediately clear that neo-Marxist theories have no potential for explaining the slow rate of implementation of RAWP. Nor, apparently, has neo-pluralist theory. Both public choice and neo-élite theories can, however, interpret this outcome as the result of defensive strategy by, respectively, managers and doctors.

Our third topic was management, where stress on management reform might be seen by neo-pluralists as aimed at securing a realignment of the various interests within the NHS, notably those at national and local levels, those involving provider groups – in particular doctors – and those providing administrative support. At a national level, government has sought through management changes to improve its grip on the NHS as a way of controlling activity within the Service more closely. The oscillation in centre–periphery relations has been a feature of the NHS since its establishment (Hunter, 1983c; Klein, 1983). Relations between the centre and the periphery have never been static; rather they are dynamic and shifting. Since the early 1970s there has been mounting concern among national policymakers over policy implementation and the so-called implementation gap. The search for better management has partly reflected the attempt by the centre to assume a more strategic directive role in relation to the NHS. However, this has been tempered by moves to devolve responsibility and encourage diversity (evident in the period 1979 to 1981 and in *Working for Patients*), which can be partially explained from a neo-pluralist perspective as an attempt to give managers more of a stake in the wheeling and dealing from which decisions on resource allocation and priorities emerge. Neo-pluralists recognize the importance of occupational politics and could explain consensus management as a device to confer status at the top table on provider groups other than the medical profession. But neo-pluralist theory offers no real explanation of why the government should wish to make these changes; in terms of the language of its proponents, why did the state need to be other than neutral on these issues?

Public choice theorists emphasize management as a means of overcoming gross inefficiency in the NHS given its position as a virtual monopoly supplier of services. They subscribe to the view that the NHS has been overadministered and undermanaged and that management consists of injecting private sector concepts into the public sector in order to secure more efficient service delivery that is responsive to consumer preferences, as expressed in the economic as distinct from the political market-place. Certainly, such concerns have been to the fore in the management reforms of the NHS. Davies (1987, p.315), for instance, argues that recent changes in the structure and management of the NHS lay the foundations 'for a new mix of public and private, statutory, voluntary and commercial services in the arena of health care delivery'. She takes issue with Klein (1984) who argues that, despite the flurry of activity, little of substance has changed; ideology may appear in manifestos but is invariably abandoned in practice.

But, whether Davies is correct or not in asserting that management reforms are a conscious attempt to follow the prescriptions of public choice theorists, most of the reforms which we have described do not, in fact, accord with such recommendations. Public choice theorists, as we noted in Chapter 1, lay great emphasis on bureaucratic empire-building as the source of public service inefficiencies, and would hardly, therefore, recommend an increase in bureaucrats' influence. The essential ingredient of public choice prescriptions is competition, and it is therefore only competitive tendering and the latest set of managerial reforms (set out in the 1989 White Paper) which accord with them. Moreover, public choice theory cannot *explain* the adoption of its own prescriptions; why 1989 rather than earlier or later? It is not especially useful in accounting for why the NHS management problem has been so pervasive under different governments nor why the solutions to it have taken the particular forms they have. Neo-élitism is probably more helpful in describing the developments described earlier that either neo-pluralism or public choice theories, but again cannot, on its own, account for them. In return for entry to the NHS in 1948, the medical profession was granted considerable autonomy in the running of the Service (Willcocks, 1967). Sections of the profession continue to occupy an influential role at local level and are also strongly – albeit less comprehensively than during the 1950s and 1960s – represented in the national policy process (see Chapter 4). The management changes documented above can, therefore, be seen as posing a threat to the supremacy of the medical profession and eroding its influence. From a neo-élitist perspective, they might, on the other hand, be seen as helping to further the interests and preferences of the medical profession. Doctors might be inclined to see improved management as a means of assisting them to utilize their resources more efficiently. They would only regard management as posing a threat if managers and professionals acting in partnership were unable to do business and were to occupy opposing camps along the lines of Alford's (1975) medical 'professional monopolists' under challenge from managerial 'corporate rationalizers'; as we show in more detail in Chapter 4 this is only very recent. An alliance between managers and professional élites is likely to become increasingly precarious if managers are seen to be, as many doctors and others already regard them, the agents not of doctors but – as a result of the strong line of accountability from the DHSS down to unit level introduced following Griffiths' proposals and *Working for Patients* – of central government (Harrison, 1988a, ch.7).

All this would amount to the development of a new, managerial, élite, easily recognizable in terms of Alford's version of neo-élitism. But again, such theories cannot *explain* the emergence of the new élite; why, despite many attempts at managerial reform, have managers only recently begun to challenge doctors?

Defining developments in management as attempts by the central state to control and regulate a monopoly service that is seen to be absorbing too many resources find considerable sympathy in neo-Marxist perspectives. Managerial reforms of the type recently witnessed in the NHS are interpreted as strategy by the capitalist state to control and contain the amount of provision offered (Davies, 1987). The need for such a strategy would derive from the failure of a capitalist economy to deliver sufficient levels of growth to enable adequate welfare state funding to be provided. From such a perspective, general management and

Working for Patients can, therefore, be seen as the start of an attempt to stimulate a mixed economy of welfare in health care, and to establish a two tier health service whereby those who can afford to exit from the NHS do so, while the public sector provides a second class service to those without the means to go elsewhere or who are categorized as bad commercial risks. Meanwhile, the rhetoric of 'efficiency' and 'cutting out waste' is seen as a device for concealing what is happening.

In some senses our conclusion to this chapter is confusing; all our four theoretical approaches are to some extent consonant with what we have described, and some even offer partial explanations; but none explains everything. The picture is further confused by the observation that some of what we have described is also consistent with the shared version that we summarized in Chapter 1; for instance the outcome of the RAWP exercise is recognizable as 'incremental politics', while a number of the changes in formal managerial arrangements are underpinned by occupational self-interest.

Yet distinctions can be made; because neo-Marxist theory is more comprehensive than the others, it offers the possibility of a more overarching explanation. And indeed, we have seen that it is the only one of our approaches which is capable of explaining the relatively sudden change in intent in managerial reforms. Yet, because of its generality, there is much that it does not explain; this suggests that there may be scope for combining it with another approach, a matter to which we return in Chapter 6.

There is, of course, a difference between the *intent* behind managerial reforms and their *outcome*. Our next chapter examines in some detail the substance of the changing relationships between managers and other groups of NHS workers.

4 The NHS workforce

In Chapter 2 we looked at financial resources in the NHS; here we turn to human resources, the cost of which accounts for almost 75 per cent of revenue expenditure (Royal Commission, 1979, p.332). Table 4.1 shows the composition of the workforce and how it has changed in the last two decades. From this, it can be seen that increases in staff have mirrored increases in expenditure; health care is a labour-intensive business with little prospect of the substitution of capital for labour. It also shows that it is *professional* staff who have been the main growth area, with manual workers declining in number. (The relatively small number of administrative and clerical staff did grow very rapidly in the aftermath of the 1974 reorganization.) In this chapter we shall be concerned with the impact of health policy on the workforce; which groups of workers have most benefitted from the organization of the NHS, and why? In order to do so, we employ Fox's (1966) distinction between 'market relations' and 'managerial relations'. Market relations are largely economic in character, centring upon the pay and other terms and conditions upon which workers are employed. Managerial relations, by contrast are political (with a small 'p') in character, and are concerned with the degree of control which the managers of an organization have over its employees. Although the distinction between the two is not absolutely watertight (for instance, industrial action in pursuit of a pay claim consists of a change in managerial relations with the intention of securing a change in market relations), we shall want to employ it in our examination of the relative treatment of different workgroups.

Specifically, we undertake four main tasks. First, we summarize the development of industrial relations in the NHS over the last twenty years, noting a considerable increase in trade union membership and activity during the 1970s. Second, we contrast this activity with its results, reaching the conclusion that there has not been any straightforward relationship between union activity and its outcomes. Third, we show that one group amongst the various groups of NHS staff has consistently fared better in respect of *managerial* relations than the others: doctors. In order to investigate this apparent élite in terms of the theoretical perspectives introduced in Chapter 1, we embark upon a fairly detailed case study of one aspect of health policy which is of profound significance to doctors themselves: the availability of consultant posts in relation to the number of junior doctors. Finally, we consider the possible implications for our analysis of the new White Paper *Working For Patients* (Department of Health et al, 1989).

Table 4.1 *Growth of the NHS workforce*

Staff group	Whole time equivalent in NHS (Great Britain)		
	1965	1975	1985
Medical and Dental	22,786	39,152	56,805
Nurse and Midwife Managers	238,705	14,204	4,949
Qualified and Trainee Nurses		287,934	375,132
Unqualified Nurses	70,579	103,679	110,904
Qualified Professional, Technical, Scientific	29,359	52,259	82,354
Unqualified Technical etc.	None	4,766	6,504
Building and Engineering Professions	2,300	6,000	7,121
Maintenance Manual Workers	19,169	23,457	24,639
Administrative, Clerical and Ambulance Officers	58,526*	109,282	135,289
Ambulance Men and Women	14,600	16,924	18,293
Ancillary	241,037	205,690	175,406
TOTAL	697,061	863,347	997,396
Non-professionals as % of total excluding Administrative etc.	54%	47%	39%

* Excludes local authority staff

Note: The figures include only salaried employees of health authorities, thereby excluding civil servants and self-employed contractors such as general practitioners. As a result of changing definitions, figures should be regarded as approximate.

Sources: *Health and Personal Social Services Statistics for England, Wales and Scotland*, various years. London: HMSO.

The development of industrial relations

At the inception of the NHS in 1948, the government had been committed to the provision of collective bargaining arrangements for its staff, many of whom had not previously been covered by such arrangements. The chosen method was to establish a number of Whitley Councils, based on a model originally proposed in 1919 in the aftermath of the First World War as a means of promoting harmony within industry generally, but never widely adopted outside the public sector. The focus of the Whitley system was at national level, with a series of joint 'functional' councils each negotiating terms and conditions for particular groups of staff. An additional general council dealt with matters common to all occupations. Provided that the relevant Minister approved them, agreements of such councils were imposed upon the NHS's component employing authorities. (For a more detailed account see Harrison, 1989.) Doctors and maintenance workers subsequently withdrew from Whitley Council coverage in favour of direct negotiations with the relevant government departments, and since 1960 the pay of the former group has been subject of annual independent review by the Review Body on Doctors' and Dentists' Remuneration (DDRB), although the recommendations of this body have not always been implemented in full by the government.

Industrial relations up to 1973 were essentially non-conflictual and national in character. Levels of trade union membership had been extremely low in the 1950s and 1960s, reaching a low point of only 32 per cent of the NHS workforce in 1966 (Barnard and Harrison, 1986, p.1218). Not surprisingly, union activity was also low, and Clegg and Chester (1957) recorded a reliance on arbitration as a means of settling NHS pay disputes, concluding that managers in industry feared trade unions much more than did their counterparts in the NHS. Moreover, this focus on industrial relations at national level meant that, although health authorities were to some extent employers in their own right, collective relations hardly existed at local level, where paternalism was the norm.

By the late 1960s, however, a number of changes had begun to occur, and, while the interrelationships between these are sometimes difficult to specify, they added up to a shift towards more adversarial behaviour and a pattern of industrial relations superficially, at least, more like that to be found in industry (Barnard and Harrison, 1986, pp.1217-20). Some of these changes were outside the NHS. Government pay policy in the late 1960s provided that productivity increases were a necessary condition of pay increases, and employment legislation after 1971 effectively required employers to introduce local procedures for dealing with such matters as discipline. Other changes were within management; as Chapter 3 noted, increasing emphasis was given to management of the NHS in the late 1960s, and this resulted in both greater specialization within management (personnel, for instance), and the introduction of quantitative techniques of work study. Other changes were within the unions. After 1970, the NHS quickly became more unionized, with some 76 per cent of workforce in membership by 1978 (Barnard and Harrison, 1986, p.1218). This trend is perhaps partly the result of economic factors (Bain and Elsheik, 1976), but also the result of competitive recruitment by some unions, for whom NHS employees provided the last large pool of unorganized labour covered by their constitutions (Klein, 1983, p.111).

By about 1970, these various factors had begun to interact; the introduction of bonus schemes for ancillary workers (such as porters, cleaners, and laundry workers) meant that *local* management–union discussions had to take place, endowing local union activity with legitimacy. Such local activism was also pursued as a matter of policy by unions such as the National Union of Public Employees (Fryer *et al*, 1974). Since managers were required by Whitley agreement to encourage employees to become union members, they found themselves unable to resist the spread of the 'check-off' of union subscriptions from employees' wages. By the mid-1970s, national agreements on the recognition of local stewards had also been reached, and local joint consultative and negotiating committees were widespread (Brand and McGill, 1978). It is important to note that these changes had spread beyond the traditional trade unions, throughout most of the professional organizations which represented NHS workers in the Whitley system. Thus, organizations such as the British Medical Association (BMA), the Royal College of Nursing, and the Chartered Society of Physiotherapy became legally registered as trade unions and began to appoint local representatives (Dyson and Spary, 1979, p.146). By the late 1970s, the unions representing ancillary and ambulance staff had begun to seek closed shop agreements (Harrison, 1988b, pp.68–70), which might be regarded as the final element in the transition of the NHS to the forms of 'mature' industrial relations found in industry.

By 1973, a major break with past practice had also occurred in terms of industrial action, with national strikes and other coercive action in support of an ancillary staff pay claim. The immediate cause of the dispute was government pay policy; a pay settlement by local authority manual workers a few days before the imposition of a pay freeze and ban on the backdating of awards had the effect of breaking a long-standing linkage without any prospect of subsequent redress. After a one day strike, action took the form of selective strikes, an overtime ban, and a campaign of non-cooperation orchestrated at local level (Bosanquet, 1979, p.7). A further national dispute (involving ancillary and ambulance staff in overtime bans and non-cooperation) took place, again in response to government pay policy, in 1978/79, the so-called 'winter of discontent'. In 1982, yet another national dispute, occurred, involving nurses, ancillaries and administrative staff, in pursuit of a 12 per cent pay claim. This dispute was marked by hitherto unprecedented inter-union cooperation, including short national strikes and a Trades Union Congress day of action (Carpenter, 1985). The years between 1973 and 1982 were also characterized by a large number of smaller disputes. Some of these were national disputes, involving smaller groups of staff; for instance, consultant medical staff treated emergencies only for a short period in 1978 (Higgins, 1988, p.69), while various groups represented by the National and Local Government Officers Association (NALGO) banned overtime in pursuit of claims over gradings and hours of work. The majority of disputes in the period were aimed at resisting planned hospital closures, while the remainder involved a range of issues concerning local management decisions; most involved ancillary staff, and some involved nurses.

Thus, over a fairly short period, an ostensibly radical change occurred in the relationships between the NHS and its staff; they became less centralized and more conflictual. But that is not to say that the *outcome* of this change was necessarily radical in terms of securing improved terms and conditions for the staff involved, and it is to this question that we turn in the next section.

The outcome of union activity: market relations

We examine the impact on market relations of changes in workforce relations described in the preceding section from three perspectives. First, we attempt to assess the outcomes of the activity in general and of the disputes themselves. Second, we examine movements in pay of NHS staff over the last twenty years, noting the origins of the most favourable awards. Finally, we note a number of recent developments in industrial relations which may be seen as indicative of contemporary power relationships in the field.

The major national disputes outlined in the preceding section can only be seen as unsuccessful from a trade union perspective, with eventual settlements differing little from pre-dispute offers (Dimmock, 1982, p.222; Carpenter, 1985). Some of the smaller disputes did, however, produce concessions; for example consultant medical staff prevented the abolition of NHS paybeds (Higgins, 1988, p.69), and maintenance electricians obtained a bonus scheme (*Health and Social Service Journal*, 29 September 1978, p.1116). Of the local disputes, those concerned to prevent hospital closures seem to have been sustainable only so long as they received medical staff support, and with one exception (the Elizabeth Garrett Anderson Hospital: Carpenter, 1985, pp.56–8) were ultimately unsuccessful. The localized management disputes are, of course, more difficult to judge, partly because of their variety and because they tend not to have been fully reported. Nevertheless, we concur with Bosanquet's judgement that many were the result of defective industrial relations procedures (1979, p.18), rather than indicative of any substantial gains for the staff. Perhaps the most that can be said is that union activity led NHS managers to be less paternal and more circumspect in their use of the 'managerial prerogative'.

Table 4.2 *Movements in salary scale maxima of selected NHS staff groups: 1965–1985 Index (1965=100)*

	1965	1970	1975	1980	1985
Medical and Dental					
Consultant	100	142	240	447	623
House Officer	100	192	336	622	877
Professional and Technical					
Highest Grade Physiotherapist	100	121	187	492	872
Basic Grade Physiotherapist	100	112	171	481	776
Nurses and Midwives					
Highest Grade Nurse Manager	100	127	321	850	1233
Ward Sister/Charge Nurse	100	129	295	565	804
Staff Nurse	100	131	311	602	819
Nursing Auxiliary	100	131	302	588	785
Administrative and Clerical					
Highest Management Grade	100	141	284	489	626
Principal Administrative Assistant	100	134	246	451	540
Clerical Officer	100	135	265	506	626
Ancillary					
Highest Male Grade	100	154	284	489	670
Lowest Male Grade	100	123	268	474	647

Source: Whitley Council Advance Letters.

Table 4.2 shows movements in the pay of selected groups of NHS staff during the last two decades. A number of observations can be made. First, professional groups have generally fared better than others. Second, differentials *within* Whitley Council groups have tended to widen. Third, despite the rapid expansion of union militancy described in the preceding section, the most favourable pay settlements have tended to occur not as a result of industrial action, but to derive from third-party reviews carried out by *ad hoc* bodies such as the Halsbury Committees on Nurses and the Professions Supplementary to Medicine (see Bosanquet, 1979, p.8). It is only occasionally that such review arrangements have been applied to ancillary staff. Where this last occurred after the 1978/79 'winter of discontent' the Clegg Commission recommended smaller awards for ancillaries (Standing Commission, 1979, p.32), who had been involved in industrial action, than for the Professions Supplementary to Medicine (Standing Commission, 1980, p.18), who had not. Moreover, when the earnings of groups of NHS staff involved in industrial action are compared with overall pay movements in Britain, it is difficult to believe that the disputes have changed very much. Figure 4.1 shows how closely ambulance staff earnings have followed the average for all males, and how closely earnings of nurses and hospital porters have followed those for all females. Finally, consultant hospital medical staff are amongst those who have fared worst in relative salary movements.

Of course, Figure 4.1 omits or conceals three other important considerations. First, it takes no account of non-pay conditions, such as holiday entitlements; these are much more advantageous to professional staff than to other groups (Barnard and Harrison, 1986, p.1221ff.). Second, it omits additional earnings from such sources as overtime, shift premia, bonus schemes and (for consultants) private patients. Finally, it conceals some rather large differences in *absolute* earnings. Thus, the average earnings of doctors are still more than three times those of trained nurses and almost four times those of nursing auxiliaries (Department of Employment, 1987).

Indeed, it was not long before the unions which represented ancillaries, and the members themselves, were to receive a more concerted battering by central government through the introduction of competitive tendering for hospital support services. (For a detailed account see Ascher, 1987.) Whereas prior to 1983 only a small proportion of services such as laundry, domestic and catering were provided by outside contractors, since 1985, health authorities have been required to let such contracts privately wherever this would result in savings. Since, in drawing up contract specifications, authorities are not allowed to specify rates of pay or conditions of employment, contracts are likely to be obtained, whether by a private contractor or by the existing direct labour force, through job losses, lower hourly rates of pay, cuts in working hours and consequent loss of the benefits of whole-time employment, and a requirement to work more intensively. Indeed, this is what has happened; although private contractors have won only a minority of contracts, such savings are said to have amounted to some £120 million per annum by 1988 (Department of Health et al, 1989).

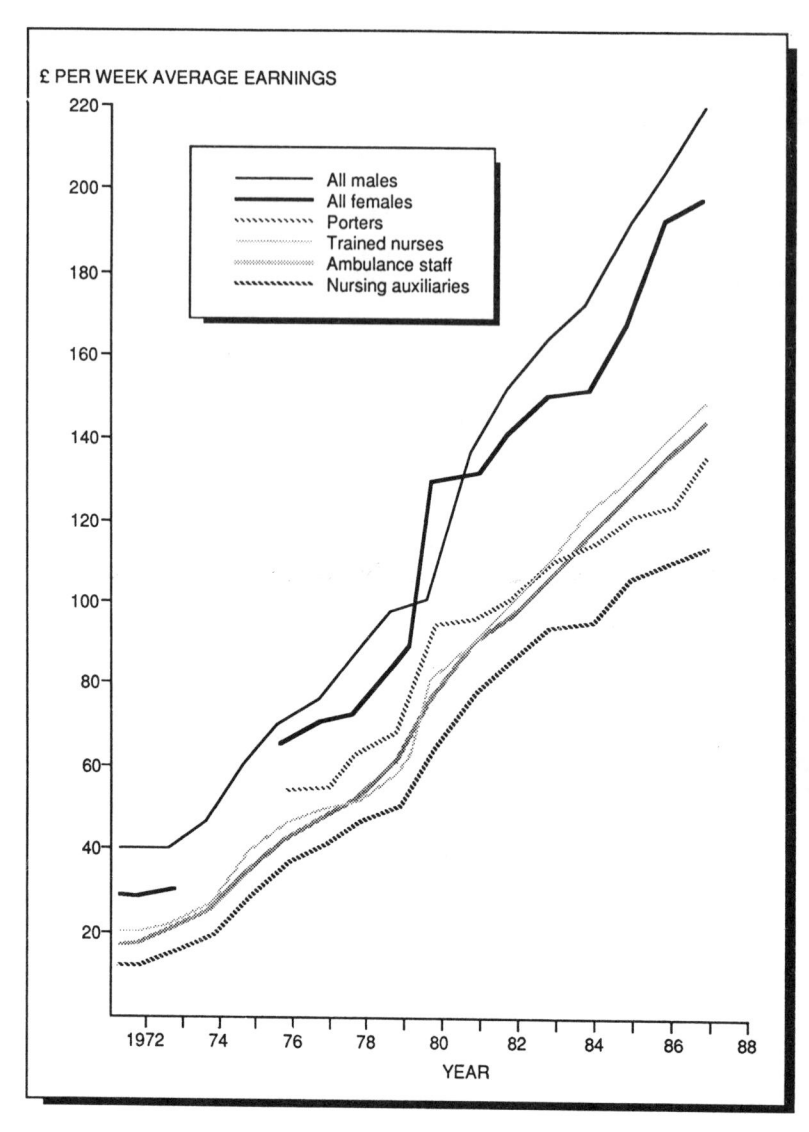

Figure 4.1 Gross pay comparisons 1972–87 in pounds per week average earnings. *Source*: Department of Employment, *New Earnings Surveys*, 1972–88, London: HMSO.

Although the response of the trade unions representing ancillary staff has been one of opposition to this development, the emphasis has been more on campaigning against the government's policy than on industrial action. For the central imposition of competitive tendering has provided a dilemma for the unions; if they oppose the process on principle, they effectively hand over the services to private contractors, but if they support tenders by the existing direct labour force, they share responsibility for worsening their members' pay and conditions. The result, therefore, has largely been for the unions to campaign against the policy on the grounds that it reduces the standard of service, and to hope (unsuccessfully, as it transpires) for public support. The unions, as organizations, have also suffered; although the National Union of Public Employees, for instance, has changed its rules in order to recruit contractors' employees, its membership levels have fallen significantly (*Institute of Personnel Management Digest*, December 1984). None of the recent spate of managerial and government initiatives outlined in Chapters 3 above have at the time of writing had comparable impact on any other staff group (Harrison, 1988c).

In summary, then, there has been little systematic relationship between the readiness of groups of NHS staff to become organized into trade unions or take part in disputes, and their relative pay. Indeed, there is an extent to which the group of staff which has been most involved in disputes, the ancillaries, has actually fared worst. The direct converse is, however, not the case; although union membership density amongst doctors is high (Certification Officer, personal communication), medical staff were involved in relatively few disputes, but have enjoyed much higher absolute earnings than anyone else; they have nevertheless lost ground in relative terms.

The pattern of managerial relations

The above picture changes quite sharply however, when managerial relations are examined, for in this area there is a clear contrast between doctors and others, though, as we shall see, this may be about to change somewhat. Despite the rapidity with which, as was noted above, the forms of mature industrial relations were adopted in the NHS, the last piece of the jigsaw, as it were, never reached its place. The unions were neither sufficiently strong nor united to obtain the closed shop agreements that they had sought, even though many NHS managers had seemed willing to negotiate seriously (Harrison, 1988b, pp.77–9).

The balance of managerial relations subsequently tipped against the non-medical staff in other ways too. Following the election in 1979 of a Conservative government, a tougher management approach to handling disputes was promulgated to the NHS in an official circular entitled *If Industrial Relations Break Down*, which exhorted managers to respond by such measures as sending staff home or reducing their pay (DHSS, 1979). And since 1983 new arrangements have been developed which remove nurses (including auxiliaries) and most other professional groups from the national Whitley system of pay negotiations, creating instead a standing Review Body analogous to the DDRB. Their pay has thus ceased to be a matter of negotiation and is instead determined by prime-ministerial decision, albeit in the light of Review Body recommendations (Harrison, 1989). Although this has so far led to larger pay awards than those received by ancillaries and others left within the Whitley system, the arrangement is likely to lead to a decline in the extent to which unions are seen to have a legitimate role. Indeed the Secretary of State for Social Services stated that any group which took industrial action could be excluded from the ambit of the Review Body (Dyson, 1983, p.996), though despite occasional industrial action in 1988 by nurses dissatisfied with the results of a national regrading exercise, this threat has not yet been carried out.

In contrast, the medical profession displays a variety of influences which have no parallels amongst other staff groups, and which are pervasive throughout the service. For instance, only doctors can refer patients to hospital or admit them when they arrive. Only doctors can prescribe drugs and refer for other treatments such as physiotherapy. Moreover, hospital consultants are often treated as having quasi-ownership of hospital beds, with the power to retain or discharge patients as they see fit; in a sense, this means that the overall shape of the services delivered by the NHS is simply the aggregate of such decisions made by individual physicians, rather than the work of politicians, planners or managers (for an extended version of this analysis, see Haywood and Alaszewski, 1980, p.304ff.). The medical Royal Colleges and Faculties play the pre-eminent role in defining medical specialties and the skills and knowledge necessary to practise within them (Harrison, 1981). Certain elements of doctors' salaries (distinction awards, which can as much as double a consultant's salary) are awarded on a confidential basis within the profession and without the involvement of managers. Nor have the latter had any right of involvement in the selection of new consultants. Finally, trading on the convention that medical knowledge is all-embracing of other varieties of health-related knowledge (Tolliday, 1978), there is pervasive medical involvement in the regulatory mechanisms for other health professions (see, for instance, Larkin, 1983). Moreover, general practitioners are self-employed, and simply unmanaged.

All these influences are linked with the notion of 'clinical freedom': that a fully qualified doctor is not subject to supervision in clinical practice, whether by a manager or by another doctor. This notion, incorporated into the culture of the NHS since its inception (for a detailed account, see Harrison, 1988a, ch.2), has served to legitimize a model of appropriate managerial behaviour as 'diplomacy'. In this model, the health service manager's role is not to lead or to change the direction of the organization, but rather to smooth out internal conflicts and to provide facilities for professionals to get on with the job of caring for patients. And indeed research carried out between the mid-1960s and the publication in 1983 of the Griffiths Report (see Chapter 3), confirms that managerial behaviour in the NHS conformed to just such a role.

According to Harrison's (1988a, ch.3) review of this research, there were four elements which contributed to the prevalence of the 'diplomat' role. First, managerial influence was not as great as that of doctors, who were not only able to exert considerable local control over specific decisions (Kogan *et al*, 1978, p.129ff.; Rathwell, 1987, ch.4; Ham, 1981, pp.147–9) but – through their 'clinically free' decisions about how to treat particular patients – determined through the aggregate of such decisions the strategic shape of services offered by the NHS (Haywood and Alaszewski, 1980, pp.104–6; Schulz and Harrison, 1983, p.33; Glennester *et al*, 1983, p.260; Stocking, 1985, pp.223–8). Second, and not surprisingly in view of the preceding factor, managerial behaviour tended to be of a problem-solving, reactive character, rather than taking the pro-active goal-seeking form dominant in managerial textbooks. This was as true of senior managers (Haywood, 1979, pp.54–7; Stewart *et al*, 1980, pp.76, 149–71; Schulz and Harrison, 1983, p.37) and planners (Barnard *et al*, 1979, vol.3; Forte, 1986, pp.24–5) as of middle managers (Harrison *et al*, 1984). Nor is there evidence of great difference outside England (Wiseman, 1979, pp.106–7).

Third, the sources of problems with which managers concerned themselves were largely *inside* the organization (Haywood, 1979, pp.57–8; Stewart *et al*, 1980, pp.170–2; Harrison *et al*, 1984). Managers were producer-oriented rather than consumer-oriented, paying relatively little attention to the views of Community Health Councils (Hallas, 1976; Klein and Lewis, 1976; Ham, 1980; Lee and Mills, 1982, p.142; Schulz and Harrison, 1983, pp.30–3) or to complaints (Thompson, 1986, p.57).

Finally, and perhaps inevitably in view of the above, the pattern of change was steady and largely incremental, with little critical analysis of the *status quo*: what we described in Chapter 1 as 'incremental politics' and 'incremental analysis' respectively (Lindblom, 1979). A major manifestation of the former was, of course, the general non-implementation of national priorities, which we discussed in Chapter 3 (see also Haywood and Alaszewski, 1980, ch.3). And incremental analysis was evident in the 'shopping list' approach to local planning adopted in both England and Scotland (Brown *et al*, 1975; Hunter, 1980).

These observations coincide quite closely with the diagnosis offered by the Griffiths Report (Harrison, 1988a, table 4.2), whose prescription was, of course, aimed at securing some change in the situation. Post-Griffiths research into NHS managers' behaviour does indeed reveal such changes; the abolition of consensus teams has been widely accepted (Harrison, Hunter, Marnoch and Pollitt, 1989a), general managers are often seen by doctors as a desirable development (Harrison and Schulz, 1988), and managers are both more cost-conscious and aware of a need to implement government policy (Harrison, 1988a, ch.7; Harrison *et al*, 1989a). But while the Griffiths changes have helped to establish greater managerial control over the professions other than medicine, evidence available at the time of writing makes it clear that there was no early change in managerial relations with doctors (Harrison, 1988c; Harrison, Hunter, Marnoch and Pollitt 1989a; 1989b).

In summary, then, the pattern of managerial relations within the NHS has to date been unequivocally biased towards the medical profession. In order to understand the nature of this bias, we need to embark upon a fairly detailed case study. For this purpose we have chosen an issue which has been recurrent over many years: the ratio of consultants to junior hospital doctors, which we examine later in this chapter.

The white paper and NHS industrial relations

Before we turn our exclusive attention to this one section of the NHS workforce, however, we want to close our general analysis of NHS industrial relations by noting that it is likely to be affected by a number of the provisions of *Working for Patients*. The most obviously important development is the proposal (see Annexe) that self-governing hospitals should be able to determine their own terms and conditions of employment (Department of Health *et al*,

1989, para.3.12), though DHA hospitals would also have some additional flexibility (para.2.18). It is difficult at present to be very confident about the likely impact of these changes on market relations, beyond noting the possibility of significant geographical variations in pay and conditions, as well as increased variation between individuals within a staff group. Competition between hospitals may exert an upward ratchet effect on pay, too. (These innovations may also affect managerial relations, as we have suggested in Chapter 3.)

But it is possible to be more confident in predicting changes in industrial relations processes. Firstly, it is likely that more managerial time than at present will have to be spent in negotiations; local flexibility implies a more-or-less constant task of negotiating *ad hoc* solutions to anomalies and leapfrogging claims. Secondly, since strikes and other service disruptions will in future entail a loss of revenue (rather than, as at present, a saving), hospitals will become, in a competitive situation, more vulnerable to industrial action than before (Harrison, Hunter, Johnston and Wistow, 1989, p.28).

Medical careers in the NHS

The career structure in NHS medicine distinguishes between career posts and training posts; the most important career posts, that is, those in which an incumbent can expect to remain permanently, are the consultant (in hospitals) and the GP. Other career posts, such as in the school medical service and hospital associate specialists are relatively few in number and, with occasional exceptions, low in status within the profession. It is therefore to consultant costs (and more recently to general practice) that young doctors have tended to aspire. Incumbents of non-career posts ('junior doctors': at present, in ascending order of seniority, house officer, senior house officer [SHO], registrar, senior registrar [SR]), are employed on fixed-term contracts of varying length and, although in reality they perform a good deal of the essential medical work of hospitals, are officially considered to be in training for career posts. It will readily be appreciated, therefore, that the ratio of career posts to training posts is potentially of crucial importance to a junior doctor; it largely determines his or her career prospects. And, as is shown below, the behaviour of junior doctors implies that the ratio is seen as important to them. Finally, the issue may also be an important one for patients, since it now seems to be widely accepted that it is preferable for them to be treated by fully trained doctors than by juniors (Social Services Committee, 1981, para.108).

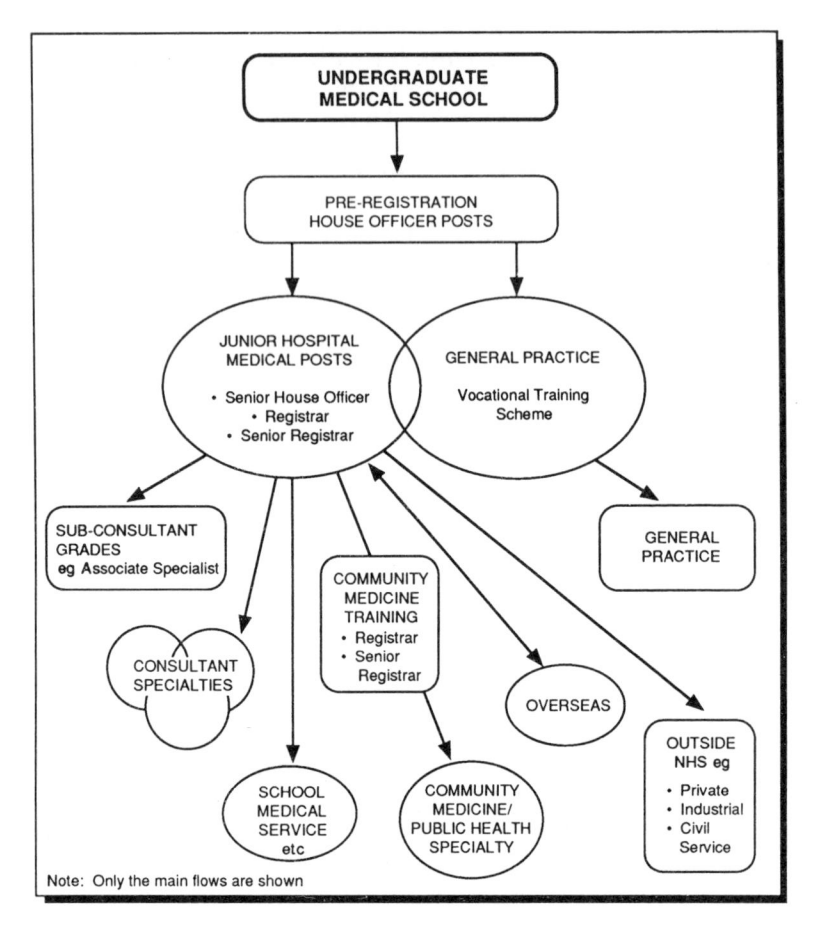

Figure 4.2 The pattern of medical careers.

Figure 4.2 provides an outline of the main flows which determine the pattern of medical careers. After graduating from medical school (usually after five years or six years), six months of hospital training is required in both a surgical and a medical pre-registration post, following which the graduate receives full registration with the General Medical Council and is legally, though not practically, regarded as able to undertake any form of medical practice. Several senior house officer posts in hospitals normally follow, as either the foundation of an intended career in hospital medicine or as part of the vocational training scheme which an aspirant to become a principal in general practice must pursue. (In the latter case, GP attachments are included.) Obtaining a post as registrar (or more particularly senior registrar) usually indicates an aspiration to consultant status. (There is a parallel arrangement for the training of the relatively small number of community physicians or public health specialists, who have consultant status but do not work in hospital.)

For those who achieve neither consultant nor GP status, there remains the opportunity of NHS employment in *locum tenens* posts, in such areas as the School Medical Service, or in a hospital sub-consultant non-training grade such as (at the time of writing) associate specialist. All these posts are relatively few in number, and do not offer either the financial rewards or status of consultant or GP. Nor are opportunities outside the NHS very significant; emigration opportunities for British doctors (especially to North America) are now much reduced by a perceived worldwide oversupply (Land, 1987), full-time posts in the civil service and industry are few in number, while the majority of private medicine is conducted on a part-time basis by doctors who also hold NHS consultant contracts (Higgins, 1988, p.52). In view of all this, it is not surprising that the vast majority of junior doctors aspire to become consultants or GPs.

Although the above account is somewhat simplified (omitting discussion of differences between specialties, the relative prospects of men and women, and geographical distribution) it is sufficient to show that the immediate determinant of juniors' chances of reaching consultant or GP status is the ratio between junior hospital medical posts and the number of consultant or GP posts, as the case may be. For much of the lifetime of the NHS, junior doctors have felt that the ratio of their own posts to consultant posts was too high to provide for reasonable career aspirations to be fulfilled and have frequently lobbied central government on these grounds (see, for instance, Eckstein, 1960; Stevens, 1966, p.145). Our case study concerns the politics of many attempts to change this ratio. But before we embark on the details, it is necessary to list the factors which, over the years, have increasingly focused attention on this ratio.

A glance back to Figure 4.2 will show that it is not, of course, only the consultant:junior ratio which determines career prospects, though a number of these other variables are at present relatively unimportant. We have already noted that opportunities in such areas as community medicine and medicine outside the NHS are relatively few, while in others such as the School Medical Service and the associate specialist grade are both few in number and low in relative status. One, more important, variable is the size of the output of medical schools, for if this were to fall then the supply of indigenous career aspirants would also fall. But this has not been the case; despite considerable controversy (Harrison, 1981, p.82), the current output of medical schools is officially seen as correct (Advisory Committee for Medical Manpower, 1985).

A second important factor is immigration; a large proportion of junior hospital doctor posts are occupied by persons born outside the British Isles, the vast majority of whom will not remain here (Smith, 1980). It is this, of course, which has sustained a higher ratio of juniors to consultants than necessary for succession planning. In 1976, some 47 per cent of junior hospital doctors were immigrants, but by 1986 this had fallen to around 31 per cent, presumably under the influence of a series of revisions to immigration rules for non-EEC graduates (Seibert, 1977, p.44; Hencke, 1985; Long et al, 1987, p.45).

The third and final important factor is the degree of availability of the major career alternative to hospital medicine: general practice. This has become both more attractive in the last twenty years, and – with the introduction of the compulsory vocational training mentioned above – more difficult to enter. It is no longer seen as the escape for those who 'fall off the ladder' of hospital careers, and decisions to pursue it now need to be taken quite soon after full registration. As Table 4.3 shows, the ratio of GPs to juniors has not been improving (from the standpoint of the career aspirant), and opportunities for entry to general practice are also restricted by the demographic structure; whereas in 1976 only 31 per cent of GPs were under forty years of age, by 1986 the proportion had risen to 41 per cent (DHSS, 1987, p.61).

Table 4.3 *Ratios of career medical posts to junior hospital medical posts, 1974–86*

Year	GPs: Juniors	Consultants: Juniors	Consultants plus GPs: Juniors
1974	1:0.78	1:1.48	1:0.51
1978	1:0.90	1:1.62	1:0.57
1982	1:0.90	1:1.66	1:0.58
1986	1:0.87	1:1.57	1:0.56

Notes: 'Juniors' as defined in Figure 4.2; GPs are defined as unrestricted principals; figures are for England.
Sources: Calculated from *Health and Personal Social Services Statistics for England*, 1982, 1985, 1986 and 1988, London, HMSO.

In summary, then, it is clear that other avenues for medical careers have not served to reduce the demand for consultant careers, while other changes, such as the reduction in immigrants willing to occupy junior posts without consultant aspirations, have merely served to increase the importance of the consultant:junior ratio, the issue to which we now turn.

The ratio of consultants to juniors: a brief history

Given that the consultant:junior ratio is, as we have shown, an important determinant of medical career prospects, it will be seen that only two strategies are available to change the ratio in favour of these prospects. Either the number of junior posts can be controlled, or the number of consultant posts increased (or both). A third possible strategy would be to sidestep the problem by the creation of an attractive sub-consultant career grade. In fact, all of these strategies have been attempted in the last forty years (some more than once) and all have failed, for reasons that we shall examine. (The evidence of failure of the first two strategies is, of course, provided by Table 4.3: the ratio has barely changed.) At the inception of the NHS, the government had wished to regard consultant grade as the sole hospital career grade, but agreed under pressure from the medical profession that career sub-consultant posts should be made available. In the event, however, it was the training grades of SHO and registrar which expanded during the 1950s, much more quickly than did career posts, with two results. First, juniors were threatened with redundancy as their fixed-term contracts expired and they were unable to obtain promotion; eventually, the Ministry of Health conceded that these grades could be regarded as career posts. Second, junior doctors began to emigrate, largely to North America and Australia; since, despite their formal status as trainees, junior doctors perform much of the medical work of hospitals, the posts had to be filled, and this was done by recruiting immigrants, often from the New Commonwealth (Watkin, 1975, p.226; Jones, 1981, p.41; Social Services Committee, 1981, para.69).

The Platt Report of 1959 responded to this situation by proposing both an expansion in consultant posts and a strategy of making the career sub-consultant grade more attractive, under the designation 'medical assistant'. Expansion of the consultant grade did occur; ministry targets were set and many sub-consultants were regraded as consultants (Shore, 1974, p.34; Appleyard, 1976, p.136). But the lack of attractiveness of the sub-consultant grade persisted and was amongst the wide range of issues addressed by the Royal Commission on Medical Education, under the chairmanship of Lord Todd, an eminent physician. Reporting in 1968, Todd proposed a fully-qualified hospital career grade of specialist, from which only some would be promoted to consultant. It was clear, however, even before Todd reported, that this was not acceptable to the BMA, and subsequent negotiations with the ministry led to a joint statement asserting the importance of the medical assistant grade. This in turn was rejected by the rank and file of BMA membership at its Annual Representatives Meeting in 1968, and a moratorium was placed on the recruitment of medical assistants (*British Medical Journal*, vol.1, 1968 suppl., pp.93–6; Shore, 1974, p.34).

In order to seek a way out of this apparent impasse, the Ministry of Health established a committee of doctors under the chairmanship of its own Chief Medical Officer; the resulting Godber Report rejected the Todd proposal, recommending instead an increase in the number of consultants, together with control of the number of junior posts. The BMA had also been considering the issue, and discussion between the ministry and the Joint Consultants Committee (JCC: the main vehicle for consultation on medical issues unrelated to pay) led in 1969 to proposals that no sub-consultant career grade should exist, and that the number of consultant posts should instead be expanded more quickly than the number of junior posts. In addition, a new grade of hospital practitioner would be created as a means of encouraging GPs to undertake part-time hospital work (Shore, 1974, p.34; Engleman, 1977, p.18), so that although 'there would no longer be a group of very experienced junior staff . . . the work of the consultant grade would not . . . be affected' (*British Medical Journal*, vol.4, 1969, suppl., pp.53–5). The health departments subsequently endorsed the illustrative figures concerned in the proposal (an annual 4 per cent increase in consultants and 2.5 per cent in juniors), expecting the two groups to be in balance by 1981.

In the event, *junior* posts grew at 4 per cent, and in 1971 there was a further joint JCC and health departments proposal: the creation of a national Central Manpower Committee (CMC) as a forum for joint discussions on medical staffing. The CMC was to consist of seventeen representatives of the profession and six of the health departments (representatives of medical education were subsequently added), and there were to be Regional Manpower Committees, consisting of local representatives of the profession, to advise health authorities. Established in 1972, the CMC (which still exists) has the power to approve proposals to create new consultant, SR and registrar posts. The CMC's first task was to secure an annual 4 per cent increase in consultant posts, through a series of regional targets, but this was only achieved in one year and the number of junior posts grew more quickly, so that (as Table 4.3 shows) the ratio of consultants to juniors continued to deteriorate throughout the 1970s. This conspicuous failure caused the 1979 Royal Commission on the NHS to revive the Todd proposals for two tiers of fully qualified specialists (Royal Commission, 1979, p.473), but this was not accepted by the government, which reiterated the policy of consultant expansion, announcing in 1981 that plans to double the number of consultants in fifteen years had been agreed with the BMA (DHSS, 1981). Concurrently, the House of Commons Social Services Committee had been considering the issue; sections of its report rejecting a sub-consultant career grade and recommending a consultant-provided service to the patient, with more consultants and less juniors (Social Services Committee, 1981, para.333) were accepted by the government (DHSS, 1982a).

Health authorities were instructed to freeze the number of SHO posts and to plan to produce a one to one ratio of consultants to juniors by 1988, and to double the number of consultants by 1996 (DHSS, 1982b, paras 3–4). Once again, however, implementation proved difficult and by 1984 the ratio still stood at 1:1.7, with no realistic prospect of reaching the 1988 target; indeed, RHAs had not even planned to reach it (*Health Service Journal*, 1 August 1985, p.952; Long *et al*, 1987, p.65).

Criticism of this failure from the National Audit Office and the Social Services Committee (Long *et al*, 1987, p.65; Social Services Committee, 1985) seems to have led to a government decision to create a new Joint Planning Advisory Committee (JPAC) with the medical profession. JPAC would devise national targets and regional quotas for junior posts (DHSS, 1985), though it was subsequently stressed that health authorities would not be compelled to create additional consultancies (DHSS, 1986).' In the meantime, discussions had been taking place between DHSS, the JCC, the Chairmen of RHAs and others (McInnes, 1987). The resulting agreement *Achieving a Balance* provided for one hundred additional consultant posts over two years, the creation of a sub-consultant career grade (subsequently entitled the staff grade), and a reduction in the number of registrar posts. The last were to be divided into posts for British (and EEC) graduates pursuing career posts and those for overseas doctors, who would be able to remain in Britain for limited periods of training only (*British Medical Journal*, vol.293, 1986, pp.147–51). The report was widely welcomed, and the new consultant posts were immediately adopted as policy. The remainder of the recommendations, and a commitment to a 2 per cent annual expansion in consultant posts were adopted as policy in 1987 (Steering Group, 1987).

It is clearly too early to make any firm assessment of whether these initiatives have been any more successful than their predecessors. Despite their apparent popularity, there have been signs that health authorities may be somewhat reluctant to seek approval for new consultants (*Health Service Journal*, 14 May 1987, p.548) and that expansion of the grade may have actually been falling, to a rate of less than 1.5 per cent annually (Millar, 1988, p.1383; *Health Service Journal*, 13 Oct. 1988, p.1183).

The politics of medical careers

Beneath this somewhat confusing account of shifting policy stances, it is possible to discern some more enduring positions adopted by each of the actors involved. Some of those will already have become obvious to the reader, others perhaps not. We can summarize them as follows.

First, junior hospital doctors wish to see a shift in the ratio in favour of more consultant posts, as an assurance against the prospect of being forced into less prestigious employment, or even, as they noted in evidence to the Social Services Committee, unemployment (Doyle, 1981). For the same reason, they do not wish to see expansion in career sub-consultant grades, a view which is perhaps held more widely in the profession (see, for instance, Shore, 1974, p.34). Not surprisingly, therefore, juniors have tended to be supporters of government policies for changing the consultant:junior ratio (Wood, 1982, p.2; *Hospital and Health Services Review*, March 1983, p.92; *British Medical Journal*, vol.293, 1986).

Second, and by contrast, existing consultants would prefer to see a lower ratio of themselves to juniors. This is to some extent a result of fears of competition over private practice (Engleman, 1978, p.3), but relates more to the recognition that juniors, despite their ostensible role as trainees, actually perform a good deal of work that would otherwise have to be undertaken by consultants. It was, for instance, this consideration that underpinned the creation in 1969 of the hospital practitioner grade. Hence, a reduction in the number of juniors implies less interesting work for consultants; the Hospital Consultants and Specialists Association (a consultants' trade union) opposed CMC policy on those grounds in the 1970s (Doran, 1973, p.72) and, along with some elements of the BMA, again in the early 1980s (*British Medical Journal*, vol.284, 1982, pp.285–6; Appleyard, 1982, p.1352). A smaller relative number of junior staff also implies a greater commitment by consultants to out-of-hours on-call duty; having themselves worked long hours as juniors, they are, not unreasonably, reluctant to continue them into middle age (Social Services Committee, 1981, paras 117ff., 235-44). Perhaps less obviously, cuts in numbers of juniors can also put at risk the continued provision of particular specialties at particular locations (Millar, 1988; Shore, personal communication, 1988).

Third, health authorities are often reluctant to seek to expand the number of consultant posts in line with prevailing government policies, and, despite the occasional threat of strong action (Social Services Committee, 1981) they have not been pressured to do so. The basis of this reluctance is related largely to finance; even where central government resources are made available for consultant expansion, they may be considered insufficient (Engleman, 1978, p.3; Social Services Committee, 1981, para. 235ff.). More specifically, the assumption is that additional consultants will take on additional work, and therefore incur considerable costs, rather than just take over existing work from juniors (Shore, personal communication, 1988). It is also unlikely that health authorities will seek to create new consultant posts without the local support of existing consultants.

Finally, governments have hitherto felt it necessary to develop policies in the area of medical staffing only with the agreement of the medical profession. The dominance of medical representation on the various committees concerned with the topic is evident from the preceding section, and what are formally consultative or advisory bodies (such as the CMC) seem often to function as negotiating forums with the health departments. But it is also evident from our account of events in the preceding section that the existence of national agreements with the medical profession has not been a guarantee of implementation. Unwillingness to impose specific consultant expansion targets on individual health authorities has allowed local interests to frustrate national policies (Ham, 1981, p.97).

Theorizing medical influence

We have seen from the first, more general, part of this chapter that medical influence is more pervasive in terms of managerial relations than of market relations. How does our case study of the politics of medical careers help us to refine this generality? To summarize the case study, governments perceive a need to reach agreement with the medical profession at national level, but neither doctors locally, nor health authorities, are bound by these agreements, and hence there has been a repeated pattern of policy statements which have failed to produce their intended results. In fact, medical manpower is by no means the only topic to which this summary might apply (Brown, 1979, p.191), though it does not apply to all policy areas (Haywood and Hunter, 1982).

In terms of the theoretical perspectives which we introduced in Chapter 1, what we have examined has some of the main features of 'liberal corporatism'. The prevalence of joint institutions for agreeing policy at national level and the monopoly of official recognition of the BMA as the only doctors' trade union are the key points here; the medical profession is deeply involved in the policymaking process. But events as described fail to meet what many theorists regard as a crucial test of corporatism (Cawson, 1985) in that the national actors have been unable or unwilling to exert discipline over those whom they represent. Local obstruction has prevailed in this as in other policy areas (Haywood and Alaszewski, 1980) and the ratio of consultants to juniors has remained much lower than intended. (It is worth noting that these observations seriously undermine general descriptions of the NHS as corporatist in character, such as that of Cawson [1982], which are presumably misled by corporatist *appearances*.)

Yet pluralist theories do not seem to offer a very close fit to the events that we have described either. Although a number of features of incrementalism, such as the evidently limited analysis of the problem of medical careers and the very slow pace of change, can be discerned, PMA was simply absent at local level, the real locus of obstruction. There were no opposing partisans and no adjustments to be made therefore; the medical profession had a local veto. Nor were the features emphasized by more recent neo-pluralist theorists very much in evidence; while representatives of junior doctors did engage in sufficient lobbying to place the matter of medical careers on policymakers' agendas from time to time, neither this nor the state acting as 'referee' has been decisive in determining the outcome.

Nor are public choice theories very helpful in explaining events; although the behaviour of the consultants in our case study can be seen as a form of personal utility maximization (that is, attempting to preserve a congenial working life), it has not, as writers such as Niskanen (1971) would predict, taken the form of budget maximization and a consequent oversupply of medical services. Neo-Marxist theories are not very helpful at our level of analysis either, since they do not have much to say about the circumstances of our case study, in which the real dynamic (or rather, static!) of events was located at micro level, and it seems difficult to hypothesize how the vital interests of the state might have been affected one way or the other by the consultant:junior ratio.

In order to find a theoretical approach which is a better 'fit' with events, we need to return to neo-élitism, but to look more broadly than liberal corporatist theories. For clearly the medical profession is an élite in the specific sense that neither governments nor managers acting on behalf of health authorities have wished to 'cross swords' with it. As the 'shared version' which we outlined in Chapter 1 emphasizes, the influence of consultants is largely defensive. But our case study enables us to go further and to suggest that this influence is located at two levels. At national level joint mechanisms ensure that policies do not radically weaken the *status quo*, but at local level consultants are often able to evade even these attenuated policies. Although, as we have seen, junior doctors have shown some ability to raise issues at national level, locally they are extremely weak, for they are employed on short, fixed-term contracts and have promotion prospects which are more than a little dependent upon references supplied by their consultants.

At national level, therefore, the appearances of liberal corporatism hold; the state eases the potential problems of regulating medical care by giving favoured status to the medical profession and involving it in joint mechanisms. But at local level, we seem to have something more akin to what Dunleavy (1981, p.13) has termed 'ideological corporatism'. The source of the consultant veto lies in the assumptions which other actors make about the consultant role; that they legitimately 'own' the services and beds that they provide, that they exercise 'clinical freedom', and that they have a monopoly of authoritative advice about service development. It is precisely such assumptions that underpin the fears of health authorities, to which we have alluded, that additional consultant posts will incur additional costs rather than taking over juniors' work.

Governments have occasionally promised to be tough on the topic of medical manpower; for instance, Patrick Jenkin, when Secretary of State for Social Services, promised strong action (Social Services Committee, 1981). But in practice, governments have been ready to pull their punches, and local managers have rarely thrown any. As Godt has noted in his comparative analysis of government/doctor relationships in three countries:

> The state seeks prior consent for its policies from providers in order to assure implementation; yet it must not give them veto power in the process (Godt, 1987, p.459).

Yet British consultants have had veto power, not just in respect of the one issue which we have examined in detail, but, as the first part of this chapter suggested, across the broad spectrum of managerial relations. In our final section we therefore attempt to assess the general implications for NHS industrial relations of *Working for Patients*.

The white paper and medical influence

We have already noted in Chapter 3 some developments proposed by *Working for Patients* which are intended to increase the potential influence of local managers in relation to doctors; more specific contracts of employment, the abolition of automatic medical representation on health authorities, and the introduction of management criteria for distinction awards are examples. But a more pervasive process of change is envisaged, for, as we have noted in the Annexe, the central assumption of the White Paper is that behaviour within the NHS can be substantially modified by the construction of a situation in which hospitals and other health care providing institutions can be made to compete against each other. The implication, therefore, is that once the new system has been established, pressures for behavioural change will be felt at *local* level; it will be upon managers that the immediate pressure of competition will fall.

In practice, hospital managers will be faced with obtaining contracts for their institutions, pricing and monitoring services, and ensuring that costs of treating categories of patients are within the revenue generated by the relevant contract. It seems clear that, under such circumstances, managers will find it necessary to revise their assumptions about the necessary legitimacy of medical decisions, and to challenge the defensive posture of the profession. We can analyse this in terms of a shift from a 'fit' with one neo-élitist theory to another. What we may be about to witness at local level is the transition from a situation which, as we have seen, resembles Dunleavy's (1981) 'ideological corporatism' to one which resembles Alford's (1975) scenario of medical 'professional monopolists' under challenge from managerial 'corporate rationalizers'. This shift from a situation characterized by a single, unchallenged, élite to one characterized by two competing élites would represent an erosion of one of the twin pillars of medical influence.

What, then, are the implications for the second pillar: medical influence at national level? Even to ask the question assumes that future governments will continue to wish to secure advance medical consent for their policies. Current evidence on this topic is mixed; on the one hand, the Secretary of State for Health has imposed a new form of contract on GPs (Moore, 1989, p.899) while on the other (to return to the topic which has occupied us for much of this chapter) he remains committed to *Achieving A Balance* and its associated joint mechanisms, and intends to fund professional education and training directly, rather than through revenue for treating patients (Department of Health, 1989a, paras 5.20–5.21). We are therefore unable to be conclusive, except to say that there is little prospect of corporatist-style NHS mechanisms disappearing rapidly. If we allow the assumption that such mechanisms will persist in the NHS, then we can predict that doctors will come to perceive them as an important means of evading local competitive pressures. To be more precise, a national agreement could be a means by which doctors attempt to resist shifts in managerial relations; a national agreement which reflected what local consultants wanted would be difficult for managers to ignore. This would not necessarily, however, enable governments to enforce national agreements which neither managers nor doctors wanted. Ironically, one effect of the White Paper may be to reinforce the community of interest of managers and consultants in maintaining the existing consultant:junior ratio.

If all or part of the costs of juniors' salaries are treated as education rather then the costs of treating patients, hospitals will (*ceteris paribus*) have an incentive to attempt to utilize them as cheap labour.

We have covered a great deal of ground in this chapter, and have already summarized at several points. In concluding it, therefore, we wish to emphasize only two points. Firstly, our analysis suggests that the proposals of *Working for Patients*, if implemented, are likely to produce significant change in the nature of medical politics. Secondly, we have suggested that, of the range of theoretical approaches introduced in Chapter 1, neo-élitism offers the best fit with our material, although in order to achieve this fit over time we have had to utilize two different theories within the broad approach. We shall return to both these matters in our concluding chapter.

5 *Measurement and evaluation*

To 'evaluate' something is to say what *value* it has – whether it is good, bad, useful, useless or any shade of these. Evaluation is seldom straightforward. Even relatively simple things like cars or houses may be assessed differently by individuals with differing viewpoints and interests. These complexities are multiplied a thousand-fold when health policies or health services are the focus of judgement. Often, the attempts to evaluate will tell the observer as much about those controlling the evaluation – about their interests and values – as about the organization or service ostensibly being evaluated.

What criteria could be used in an evaluation of, say, the NHS? One does not have to be an expert evaluator to assemble quite a long list of possible candidates. First there is the question of *effectiveness*; that is, does the NHS achieve what it was set up to achieve? Crudely, does it cure people, at least where cures are technologically possible, and does it alleviate things for those suffering pain and distress? Even this first question is extremely difficult to formulate precisely, let alone answer, because it presupposes that what the NHS is intended to achieve is fairly clear and well specified. Many commentators, both academic and practitioner, have noted that this is not in fact the case. Indeed, as we showed in Chapter 3, a major problem in recent years has been the lengthening list of 'priorities' on top of the usual (and familiar) priority care services: AIDS, waiting lists, coronary by-pass operations, cervical cancer screening services, breast cancer screening. There is actually a long history of debate about what the NHS's priorities should be; the alternative possibilities of care, cure and prevention are neither mutually compatible nor, in practice, pursued with anything like equal vigour.

Closely related to the concept of effectiveness is that of *quality*. This term is used in a wide variety of ways, but the way it will be used here is to denote *how appropriately a particular feature of the care process is carried out*. Thus, all surgeons sometimes make mistakes but, for a given type of case, a high quality surgeon makes fewer than an average surgeon. Both may be effective, in the sense that most of their operations are successful (there is no question of general incompetence) but the high quality surgeon is slightly more effective in a slightly higher proportion of similar cases. The same notion could be applied to, say, a hospital receptionist. The average receptionist may manage to help and/or reassure 70 per cent of the people who present themselves at the desk. Outstanding receptionists may do the same for 80 per cent – they are even more effective than their 'average' counterpart. Notice therefore, that 'quality' is a feature of health care *processes* as well as *outcomes*; in this sense it is a broader (some would say looser) notion than effectiveness, and concerns non-clinical as well as clinical aspects of care. High quality care is 'appropriate' in the sense that it meets the needs and wishes of the consumer. This idea of 'fitness for purpose' therefore opens up the question of *whose* purposes are to count, and since the mid-1980s much of the debate on 'quality' (at least in Britain) has been concerned with enhancing the influence of the consumer.

A second fairly obvious criterion is that of *efficiency*. Strictly, this is a ratio measure – the ratio between resource inputs (including staff) and service outputs (number of cases treated, vaccinations given, screenings carried out, and so on). If a greater output can be achieved for the same input, or the same output for a reduced input, or the ratio increased in any other way, then an increase in efficiency has occurred. Efficiency is thus distinct from *cost-effectiveness*, since the latter is a ratio between inputs and results achieved (impacts, outcomes) rather than between (as with efficiency) inputs and services provided (outputs). A completed coronary artery by-pass graft operation would be an *output*, the patient's increased life expectancy an *outcome*.

A third criterion might be the *responsiveness* of NHS services to the needs of its 'customers'. Because customers' needs are so various, so could be the actual measures adopted to try to capture 'responsiveness'. One might, for example, want to know how long people with specified conditions had to wait for hospital treatment. Or how adequate was the transport to carry people who could not carry themselves between their homes and their places of treatment. Or whether hospital patients found the food palatable. Or whether receptionists were perceived as helpful or insensitive. Or whether doctors and nurses took the trouble to explain to patients the nature of their conditions and what was being done for them.

Fourth, since *equity* was an important consideration for many of those who set up the NHS, there is obviously a case for developing measures to help monitor the distribution of NHS services between different locations and between different social groups as defined by the major lines of cleavage in our society, i.e. social class, gender, race and age. Are some groups getting a poorer service than others, relative to their needs? Furthermore, if equity is to be defined as the receipt of a fair share according to need, who is to define 'need'?

Many other criteria could be added, but these four, which are summarized in Figure 5.1, seem important enough and sufficiently representative of the difficulties of measurement and evaluation to serve as the basis for the discussion in the remainder of the chapter. Our main purpose will be to assess how and how far attempts have been made to measure effectiveness, efficiency, responsiveness and equity, and how the results of any such attempts may have influenced the policy process.

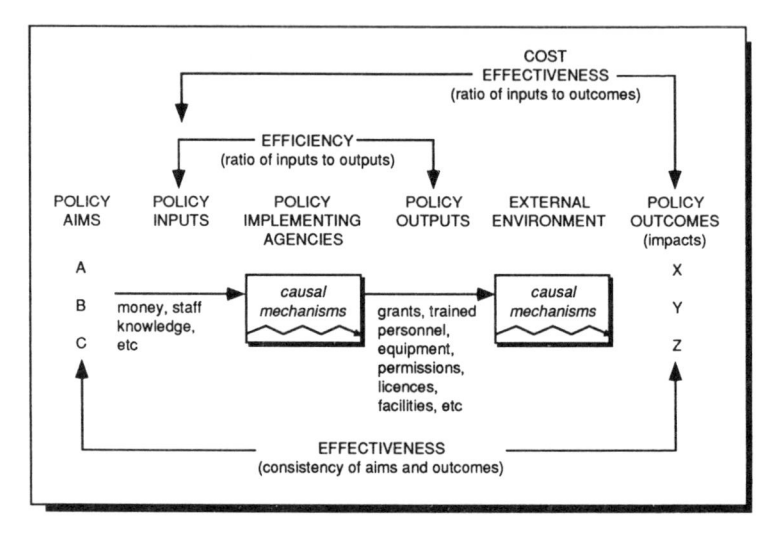

Figure 5.1 Evaluation of concepts.

Power and evaluation

Before discussing what has actually happened it may be illuminating to return to the four theoretical perspectives introduced in the first chapter. What would each of them predict about the nature and extent of evaluation in the NHS? Subsequently these predictions can be compared with what is known of recent and current practice.

The reader should, however, be warned that none of the theories concerned was 'purpose-built' to generate predictions of this kind. They are, as was explained, theories principally concerned to analyse the broad distribution of power in our societies and their major institutions. The following exercise is therefore somewhat speculative and interpretive. The neo-pluralist perspective would certainly not encourage its users to expect to find a rational and/or comprehensive system of careful measurement and evaluation of either NHS services or (more generally) the impacts of governmentally enunciated health policies. Neither would any of the other three perspectives introduced in Chapter 1. All would expect the unequal distribution of power in health care policymaking to be reflected not merely in the policies themselves but also in the ways in which these policies were judged.

Neo-pluralists might well expect there to be an on-going argument about what evaluation should be conducted, with the principal power groupings each seeking measures which would minimize the exposure of their own arrangements and resource position to public criticism. Government would have an important role in seeking to limit this potential cacophony by emphasizing the broad public interest, and its own interest as paymaster to the NHS. Thus one might see government pushing for measures of efficiency and cost-effectiveness (what is achieved per unit of resource input) and the medical profession and other provider organizations advocating instead measurement of population health needs and of growth in services, both of which would be likely to indicate the need for *more* provision. One area where the government efforts would be least likely to make headway, however, would be in the development of measures of the efficiency and cost effectiveness of major private sector suppliers and providers. Thus one would not expect it to be easy to get systematic information on these counts about pharmaceutical supplies to the NHS or about the relative efficiency and effectiveness of private versus NHS hospitals and clinics. Another area where progress could be expected to be slow would be in the establishment of any clear official statement of the priorities of the NHS. Neo-pluralists would tend to believe that the constant juggling for position between interest groups with rather different priorities would make it hard to get agreement on a single statement of priorities. Even if government were willing to risk putting its authority behind such a statement the neo-pluralist perspective would predict difficulties in carrying those expressed priorities into actual practice. It is interesting, in this regard, that the first real attempts at such a statement did not appear until the NHS was nearly thirty years old (DHSS(NI), 1975; DHSS, 1976; Welsh Office, 1976; Scottish Home and Health Department, 1976).

Public choice theorists, since they predict persistent oversupply of monopoly and near-monopoly public services, would expect the service providers such as doctors to collude with sympathetic politicians and bureaucrats in concealing the extent of the inefficiency in the existing arrangements for the NHS. Public choice theorists would also anticipate only weak development of measures of consumer responsiveness for very much the same reasons. Monopolists, according to this theory, simply do not have to pay as much attention to consumer wants as providers who compete with each other in a market. The only type of measure which the monopoly providers and their colluding bureaucrats would be relatively keen to see established would be professionally defined measures of *need*, rather than performance. Measures of need would help providers sustain their continuing demands on government for increased resources.

Neo-élitists would share many of the predictions of the two preceding perspectives, but would adopt a slightly different emphasis in explaining how strong effectiveness or efficiency or responsiveness measures are avoided. They would tend to see the medical profession as being in the driving seat, and the division between the public and private sector as less important than the underlying élite unity of the doctors. In the liberal corporatist version of élite theory, performance measures would appear as unwanted because of their potentially disruptive effects on the close relationship between the medical profession's peak associations and the DoH. Only if the profession in some major sense 'failed to deliver' (as, for example, Chapter 4 suggested they had done in respect of controlling rank and file consultants over the junior: senior ratio) would the DoH be driven to try to impose its own forms of control – which might well include evaluation of the efficiency and effectiveness of medical practice. Until such a breakdown in élite accommodation, however, one would expect evaluative procedures to be left firmly in the hands of the profession itself, and therefore to be largely concealed from public view. An obvious example of this kind of arrangement would be the system of 'merit awards' through which allegedly meritorious consultants are awarded considerable salary increases. The selection criteria for these awards have always been vague and obscure and the actual process of selection both confidential and wholly under the control of senior consultants themselves. Indeed, from a neo-élitist perspective these awards could be seen, historically, to originate as government 'bribes' to help persuade hospital doctors to join the NHS.

The neo-Marxists would probably have little to say about evaluation, at least in any detailed sense. Given their emphasis on the class structure of capitalist society they might predict that the dominant class would be anxious to minimize spending on the

NHS ('socialized medicine') just as they would seek to restrain all 'social consumption' expenditure because of its predominantly negative effect on capital accumulation. (For the distinctions between social expenses, social consumption and social investment, see Chapter 1.) Therefore one could expect the greatest government efforts to go into establishing measures of economy and efficiency. Policy would in practice reflect the status of the NHS as a kind of 'necessary evil', part of the welfare provision that helped to legitimize the state and disguise its customary pro-capitalist, anti-worker bias. Marxists are therefore unsurprised to find large gaps between the official rhetoric of a first class health service, available to all, and the actual practice of penny-pinching economy drives, encouragement of private practice (at least under the Conservative administration from 1979) and a failure to measure and locate the real sources of sickness (the exploitative nature of capitalist relations). A genuine drive to measure and increase effectiveness would inevitably begin to track down these unpalatable aspects of the larger social system, and would therefore hardly be likely to rank high on the stage agenda; the attempted suppression of the 'Black Report' on inequalities in health might be cited as evidence of this (Townsend and Davidson, 1983, pp.11–12). A more attractive strategy for a capitalist state, neo-Marxists might argue, would be to blame the victims of ill health. If it could be suggested that fecklessness and self-neglect were the principal causes of sickness, then the burden of change could be thrown onto the workers rather than the capitalists.

The evaluation of NHS services: a brief history

In a sense, this could be a very brief history because there is so little – until recently – to record. It remains the case, for example, that across very broad areas of NHS activity there is no direct assessment of the extent of cure or care or improvement achieved. Indeed, it was not until the late 1980s that many hospital record systems began to distinguish between deaths and discharges. In 1988 a National Audit Office study concluded that: 'whilst fully recognizing its importance, the DoH had still to agree a national strategy for ensuring the effectiveness of clinical care,' and that the Welsh Office and SHHD were little further forward (National Audit Office, 1988, pp.1–2). Nor is there any routine monitoring, either by the employer or by the profession, of the competence of individual GPs or consultants. The same National Audit Office study observed that:

The professions actively influenced the standards of health care in a number of ways, but there was an absence of comprehensive monitoring arrangements and clinicians were not expressly required to evaluate effectiveness (National Audit Office, 1988, p.1).

This lack of any comprehensive evaluation of effectiveness is not simply due to professional or departmental reluctance. For it has also long been recognized that the effectiveness of many standard medical procedures is unproven – and hard to demonstrate (Cochrane, 1972). In what is now regarded as a classic essay on the evaluation of medical care the then Director of the Medical Research Council's Epidemiology Unit wrote that there were 'strong suggestions of inefficient use of therapies, and considerable use of ineffective ones' (Cochrane, 1972, p.67). As the 1979 Royal Commission on the National Health Service put it: 'Medicine is still an inexact science, and many of the procedures used by doctors, nurses and the remedial professions have never been tested for effectiveness' (Royal Commission, 1979). Furthermore, in so far as effectiveness has been thus entrusted to the medical profession it should be borne in mind that, throughout the period under consideration:

> The English doctor who is not in a training grade is in many ways more independent than his (sic) American counterpart. The consultant receives, in effect, a lifetime appointment . . . The GP has independent contractor status, but unlike most contractors his performance is not reviewed periodically (Fox, 1978, p.10).

It would be misleading, however, to leave the impression that there is absolutely no monitoring for quality or effectiveness. There are many local, internal monitoring procedures run by particular medical departments in particular hospitals. These are invariably closed to the public view. More important, following a major scandal at Ely geriatric hospital, the DHSS created in 1960 a quasi-inspectorate, entitled the Hospital Advisory Service. In 1976 it was renamed the Health Advisory Service (HAS) and its writ was extended to community services and long-stay facilities for children (DHSS, 1977). The HAS sends teams of consultants, nurses, therapists, managers and Social Services inspectors into these facilities on a cyclical basis. Each district may expect to be visited once every eleven or twelve years. The resulting report goes to the DHA concerned. Initially these were confidential, but since 1985 they have been published.

How effective has the HAS been? The authors of a recent review comment that:

> HAS advice is precisely that: advice. Its reports carry no mandatory force. They are exercises in persuasion, whose force largely depends on the professional authority of the visiting team (Day, Klein and Tipping, 1988, p.40).

Local reactions to HAS advice have varied considerably. Some DHAs respond vigorously, and in detail. Others appear to be both vague and very cautious about the extent to which they are willing and able to change their practice. Overall, it is clear that:

> The remit of the HAS is limited to services for the most deprived groups: it provides no information about the performance of the NHS as a whole. In part this may reflect the anxiety of central policy-makers to have information about the most scandal-prone sectors of the NHS, where clients tend to be exceptionally vulnerable and therefore in need of protection. However, it also reflects the fact that these are the sectors of the NHS which come near the bottom of the medical profession's own hierarchy of prestige, and where doctors, indeed, tend to play a less dominant role than in the acute services. The profession as a whole, therefore, did not see the introduction of the HAS as a direct attack on medical acute autonomy (Klein, 1982b, p.398).

The situation with respect to *responsiveness* is not very different. The Griffiths team, in its diagnosis of NHS problems in the early 1980s, commented that 'Businessmen have a keen sense of how well they are looking after their customers. Whether the NHS is meeting the needs of the patient, and the community, and can prove that it is doing so, is open to question' (NHS Management Inquiry, 1983). Four years later Sir Roy Griffiths, by this time special adviser to the Prime Minister on health policy, was still saying 'I actually believe that a lot more can be done within the NHS, accepting that it is a monopoly provider, to ensure that the consumer is better looked after' (Griffiths, 1987, p.88). Between these two dates a large number of 'consumerist' initiatives had been spawned, but many of them had a rather superficial, 'charm school' air about them, and few appeared either to empower the consumer with genuine choice or to trespass on the sacred turf of doctors' discretion and clinical freedom (Pollitt, 1987; 1988). *Equity*, at least in the geographical sense, did begin to receive significant policy attention in the early 1970s, culminating in the adoption of the RAWP formula (see Chapter 2) in 1976. Equity as between social classes, ethnic groups, men and women, and people of different age groups has been a focus of academic research since the early 1970s, but does not appear to have embedded itself much in the policy process, at least not at national level. For the first quarter century or so of the NHS's existence the widespread assumption seems to have been that the fact that its services were open to all and free (apart from prescription charges) at the point of access was sufficient to guarantee equity.

The measurement of *efficiency*, however, provides rather a different story. The NHS was less than ten years old when its costs (inputs) first became the subject of a major public investigation. The Guillebaud Committee reported in 1956 that the NHS was not guilty of extravagance or inefficiency. Certainly NHS expenditure had quickly exceeded the government's original estimates, but those estimates had been erected on the unrealistic assumption that the NHS would soon begin to reduce the total quantity of sickness in the community, and that its costs would therefore fall. Furthermore, much of the apparent increase in expenditure was due to general price inflation and in terms of its share of GNP the cost of the NHS had actually fallen from 3.75 per cent in 1949/50 to 3.25 per cent in 1953/54 (Committee of Enquiry, 1956).

Guillebaud proved to be the first of many investigations and exhortations concerning expenditure. Like Guillebaud, many of these did not manage to get to grips with efficiency in the full sense, but concentrated mainly on *economy* (costs) – the input half of the efficiency ratio. When, in 1977, the Parliamentary Select Committee on Expenditure turned its attention to the issue of how 'increasing expenditure has, over the years, been reflected in the services concerned' (i.e. output: Expenditure Committee, 1978) it found that the available official statistics were inadequate for this task. Other committees subsequently came to broadly similar conclusions, culminating in a particularly critical attack on the deficiencies of the DHSS's monitoring by the Public Accounts Committee in 1982 (Committee of Public Accounts, 1982; see also Klein, 1982b, pp.399–403).

From about this time – the early 1980s – a step change in the total amount of monitoring and evaluation is discernable. This more intensive stage will be dealt with in greater detail in the next section. It is worth pausing at this point, however, to note that the brief history thus far does indeed appear consonant with at least some of the main expectations generated by adopting a 'distribution of power' perspective. None of our four power theories would predict great efforts being invested in the evaluation of either overall NHS effectiveness or the quality of care provided by individual doctors . And that is exactly what the historical record discloses. All, except public choice theory, would predict that such efforts as might be essayed would be focused on issues of economy and efficiency rather than effectiveness, responsiveness or equity. And the shrewd user of public choice theory might point out that, although there has been much *talk* about efficiency, especially of late, it is far from clear that this has changed much medical *behaviour*. In any event the proposed primacy of concern for economy and efficiency does appear to have been the case (though with the partial exception of geographic equity) at least from the early 1970s. It remains to push the application of these theories further, and in particular to see if it is possible to distinguish between their respective explanatory powers. This interpretive task will be addressed in the final section of this chapter, after a more detailed examination of recent developments.

From the early 1980s there developed a veritable rash of new monitoring and evaluation schemes, initiated mainly by the DHSS, but with some echoing, independent responses from professional bodies and consumer groups. It is impractical to attempt a comprehensive listing here (especially since the national initiatives soon stimulated many local variants and experiments in individual health authorities) so instead a selection will be made, and the selected schemes subjected to further discussion.

The basis of our selection is as follows. First, we have included all the major national schemes of monitoring and evaluation applied to all English health authorities (some variations between countries being noted). Second, we have added two of what we judge to be the most interesting and innovative schemes developed by professional bodies (for a more extensive listing of these, see Shaw, 1986). Third, we have also included a brief discussion of one attempt by a consumer group to move into systematic monitoring activities, and a summary of public opinion concerning the Service. Taken together, this selection produces the sequence shown in Table 5.1.

The review process

The review process is conceptually so simple that the only surprise is that it took until 1982 to arrive at it. In England the basic idea is that each layer in the NHS (RHAs, DHAs, units) should have objectives, and plans to achieve those objectives, and

Table 5.1 *Key developments in evaluation, 1980–9*

1982	Annual ministerial reviews of RHAs, with parallel RHA reviews of DHAs (no Scottish equivalent)
1982	Introduction of 'Rayner scrutinies' to the NHS
1983	First national performance indicator package produced by DHSS (no Scottish equivalent)
1984	DHA reviews of units
1984	Association of Surgeons and Association of Anaesthetists set up Confidential Enquiry into Perioperative Deaths (CEPOD)
1984	College of Health (consumer group) publishes first issue of *Hospital Waiting Lists*
1985	Royal College of General Practitioners publishes *What sort of doctor? Assessing quality of care in general practice*
1985	Improved packages of performance indicators (PIs) issued by DHSS (still no PIs in Scotland)
1986	Annual performance reviews of regions by NHS Management Board
1987	Individual performance review (IPR) and performance-related pay (PRP) introduced for general managers
1987	CEPOD report published (Buck *et al*, 1987)
1987	Government publishes White Paper on primary care *Promoting Better Health*, including proposals for incentives for good practice and support for peer review experiments (DHSS *et al*, 1987)
1989	White Paper *Working for patients* includes proposals for medical audit (peer review) among both consultants and GPs. Also responsibility for the external audit of both health authorities and FPCs is to be transferred from the DoH/Welsh Office to the Audit Commission. In Scotland, however, the SHHD remains responsible

that once a year the layer above will formally check the progress (or lack of it) with those plans. It is a tribute to the highly decentralized character of the service that it was not until 1982 that such a checking procedure was put in place, and that it then immediately became the focus for suspicions of 'centralization' and 'political control'.

The review process has gone through a number of changes since it was introduced. At its inception, stress was laid on the personal participation of ministers in annual meetings with RHA chairpersons. No doubt this reflected the immediate circumstances of the time – the Public Accounts Committee had just issued a strong criticism of the DHSS's lack of control over manpower and the commissioning of new hospitals (Committee of Public Accounts, 1981; Harrison, 1988a, p.102). Equally significant, however, were the parallel reviews of DHAs by their RHAs and the conscious move away from the previous style of centre-local planning which had depended heavily on the production by the

DHSS of an endless stream of health circulars and consultative documents. From 1984 district reviews of units were added to the cycle, and in 1986 *performance* reviews of regions were put in place alongside the continuing ministerial reviews. As one of the architects of performance reviews explained:

> Annual reviews [i.e. ministerial reviews] have concentrated on the longer term strategic elements in policies and plans rather than on the equally important short term aspects of service delivery . . . One of the central aims of the new performance reviews was to plug this gap (Mills, 1987, p.470).

This new element in the review process was carried out not by ministers, but by the NHS management board. It focused not only on the substantive short term issues of 'cost improvement' programmes and service developments, but also on the effectiveness of regional systems for monitoring districts. The distinction between ministerial reviews and performance reviews was evidently a necessary one in the light of early experience with ministers who found it difficult to comprehend the full complexity of the review process.

One can therefore see in the development of the review process a movement from departmental monitoring of broad strategies to deep monitoring of short term operational plans and of control systems stretching right down to unit level. Furthermore this took place during a period when the centre had increasing resort to earmarked funding of particular programmes, many of which sported their own elaborate monitoring requirements. The combined effect of all this was, at minimum, a much denser network of accountability. As one dispirited regional officer put it to us early in 1988: 'There are people in London whose aim in life is to present reports to the NHS management board. Those reports could be about the price of fish.' Arguably, however, it meant more than this – it signified an unprecedented increase in central control. Interestingly, the 1989 White Paper claimed that, with the creation of a policy board and a management executive it introduced 'for the first time a clear and effective chain of management command, running from Districts through Regions to the Chief Executive and from there to the Secretary of State' (Department of Health *et al*, 1989b, p.13). But to what kind of evaluation was this tighter control directed? In the main it was directed at economy, efficiency and conformity to plans. During the 1980s, at least, the review process seldom directly addressed questions of effectiveness or responsiveness.

Performance indicators

At the same time as the review process appeared on the scene, the DHSS also introduced a set of national 'performance indicators' (PIs). In the autumn of 1983 each of the 192 DHAs and 14 RHAs received a statistical package, prepared by the DHSS, which comprised up to 147 individual indicators. Each indicator was a quantitative measure of some aspect of clinical activity, finance, manpower, support services or estate management. Examples of the most often cited clinical indicators included the average length of stay in hospital by medical specialty, the average number of patients per bed per year ('throughput'), and the number of in-patient admissions per thousand population served by the district in question. Using these indicators, districts could compare their 'performance' with those of other districts in the same region, or indeed, with the national average.

This scheme was introduced in some haste, partly – like the review process – to cover ministerial flanks against telling Parliamentary criticism (Pollitt, 1985a). It was not, at first, clearly linked to other, on-going NHS processes of planning or resource allocation. In some places it did feature as a distinct item in regional reviews of districts, but in others it seemed at first to be a free-standing exercise, and one lacking any particularly potent penalties or incentives. Early research seemed to show that only a minority of consultants took much notice of it, and even fewer Community Health Councils (CHCs) (Pollitt, 1986a). The indicators themselves fell mainly into the economy, efficiency and process categories – few of them were directly assessed outputs or outcomes (Pollitt, 1986b). Most of the data were well over two years old, and there were widespread complaints (even from those who supported the exercise in principle) about frequent inaccuracies (Pollitt, 1986a). Subsequently, however, considerable improvements were made. In 1985 a second, and then a third set of PIs were issued. These covered more services (the first set had been very hospital-centred), were more up-to-date, somewhat more reliable and much more 'user-friendly' in their presentation (they used computer graphics instead of columns of figures in hard copy). Despite these real gains, however, the fundamental limitations of the exercise remained. There were still very few indicators of outcomes, and therefore of effectiveness. Family practitioner services were still excluded from the exercise. The relevance of many of the indicators to specified policy objectives was far from clear. A start was made on including measures of the 'acceptability' of certain services, but consumers (patients and potential patients) played no part in the definition of this concept (Pollitt, 1985b).

During 1987, a substantial independent research programme was carried out to establish what was being made of PIs, and how they were regarded (Jenkins *et al*, 1987). The findings were mixed, in the sense that, although it was clear that PIs were regularly referred to by district general managers, planners and information specialists, the limitations associated with the very first (1983) PI package were still visible. Only a minority of the consultants, CHCs and nurses interviewed appeared to be active 'users'. Many of those who did use the PIs had problems comprehending them: 'Some users were able to consider the inter-relationship of several PIs at once and appreciated the fact that they can rarely be used singly, but this skill was only seen in a small percentage of users' (Jenkins *et al*, 1987, p.149). In conclusion the study warned that 'Massive investments in the technical qualities of PIs may not yield much if local managers do not trust them, or have no way of integrating them into local performance evaluation' (p.5). In sum, therefore, the PI system bears the appearance of a centrally driven exercise which has focused on efficiency far more than any of our other three evaluative criteria (effectiveness, responsiveness, equity). Despite their title, PIs have not penetrated very far at all into the realms of the success or otherwise of cure and care. Neither have they commanded much attention from the medical profession, or from consumers. Nothing has yet happened fundamentally to disturb the judgement made when the impact of the first PI package was investigated: that it was a 'top-down' initiative, and one apparently embarked upon for a restricted audience and without a clear view of its full implications. Few new resources were invested in it, and no new incentives created (Pollitt, 1986a, p.456).

Rayner scrutinies

Rayner scrutinies, like ministerial reviews, were introduced in 1982. They are not a country-wide system like PIs or the review process, but rather a particular technique for producing quick, highly focused reviews of particular services and for ensuring that something then gets done about the review's recommendations. The scrutinies were named after Sir Derek (later Lord) Rayner, who was 'borrowed' from Marks and Spencer by Mrs Thatcher in 1979 to examine the efficiency of the public sector. The early scrutinies were conducted mainly in the civil service (for a case study see Warner, 1984), but soon they came to be applied to the NHS as well. The key features of most of these scrutinies were fivefold. First, they carried considerable clout. Lord Rayner was known to be close to, and much admired by, the prime minister and most of the scrutiny reports, were directly monitored by No.10. Second, the principal aim was to increase efficiency. 'Savings' were the major currency of most of the scrutinies. Third, the method by which the review was carried out was relatively novel, both for Whitehall and the NHS. Instead of setting up some sort of more-or-less representative committee, scrutinies were usually given to individual officers (often quite junior, but well regarded – Clive Ponting was one of the early 'young Turks' of scrutineering) or, at the most very small teams. Fourth, the time scale for completion was rapid by normal bureaucratic standards – usually ninety days. Finally, procedures were established for ensuring immediate attention to the report at the highest official implementation of any decisions reached on the basis of the scrutineers' recommendations.

Taken together, therefore, these characteristics made Rayner scrutinies rapid, high-powered ways of getting things changed in the cause of efficiency. In the NHS scrutinies were carried out, for example, on the ambulance service, community care in Wales, and income generation (see Harrison, 1988a, ch.4 for details). They are a further example of the Conservative government's prime concern with economy and efficiency, and of their willingness to impose new monitoring devices on health authorities.

Professional initiatives

The Confidential Enquiry into Perioperative Deaths (CEPOD) was a very different kind of exercise. It was mounted by the medical profession (the Association of Anaesthetists and the Association of Surgeons, jointly) and was careful to stay clear of any DHSS participation, or even sponsorship. The aim was not principally efficiency, but rather the effectiveness and quality of inpatient surgery. CEPOD arose because of the concern of some senior surgeons and anaesthetists at the results of two previous enquiries, one into bowel cancer and one into the mortality associated with anaesthesia. These and other studies were making it increasingly clear that there was very considerable variance in perioperative mortality rates for the same condition treated in different places or by different surgeons. Consultants in health authorities which volunteered to participate in the CEPOD study had to fill in carefully designed forms which asked for details of the circumstances surrounding every surgery-related death within thirty days of an operation, and of the medical procedures performed. These forms were than analysed by a national team of expert (consultant) assessors. An elaborate system of anonymously coding the forms ensured that even the assessors did not know whom they were assessing.

The CEPOD report was published at the end of 1987 (Buck et al, 1987). To avoid possible legal action the survey data were protected by crown privilege and destroyed as soon as the analysis on them had been completed. The report did not find any dramatic, single cause of avoidable deaths, but did identify a number of worrying practices and variations. For example 'Our assessors are . . . concerned that many operations are undertaken by surgeons too junior or too inexperienced to do the job'. Or 'General surgeons doing non-urgent brain surgery . . . and orthopaedic surgeons doing bowel surgery are examples that are difficult to defend'. There were also comments on equipment shortages and over-tight operating schedules.

CEPOD was thus an example of the profession voluntarily monitoring its own quality of practice. The report gained little publicity in the national press or on television; ward closures and nurses' discontents which were occurring at the same time commanded much more popular attention. Participation by individual doctors was entirely voluntary. A small number refused to take part, or effectively dropped out with the result that 13 per cent of the 4,034 registered deaths could not be assessed (Devlin, 1988, p.312). Furthermore, even in those (rare) cases where the enquiry found evidence of possible individual incompetence, the surgeons and anaesthetists concerned were protected by the strict confidentiality of the whole exercise. Management could take no case-specific remedial or disciplinary action, although they could, of course, pursue the general lessons of the report.

In *Working for Patients* the government expressed enthusiastic support for the principle of peer review. Not only was CEPOD to be extended (with departmental support) but the government declared its intention of working with the profession to set up a medical audit committee in each district. Although the government's wording emphasized that this would be a matter for the profession, there was also a hint of management 'closing in' on clinical quality and effectiveness. For although doctors were to conduct the audits, management was said to have a responsibility for seeing that suitable audit procedures were indeed put in place. Furthermore it was suggested that at least the general tenor of the findings of local audits should be made available to local management (Department of Health et al, 1989b). At the time of writing it remains to be seen exactly how these proposals will be put into effect, and how much local variation in the practice of audit will be tolerated. In these respects the 1989 White Paper could represent anything from a modest, incremental step towards improved quality control to a quite radical incursion on medical autonomy.

Thus far in this chapter little has been said about primary care. Our silence is partly a function of how little work has been done to evaluate the services offered by GPs and their teams. After reviewing what *was* known, Maynard (1986, p.197) concluded:

> Not only is general practice an uncharted jungle, its interface with other parts of the NHS is such that incentives at the margin induce inefficiency, with the cash-limited hospital services . . . trying to shift costs onto the open-ended primary care service and vice versa.

In 1975, however, the Royal College of General Practitioners (RCGP) published a report *What Sort of Doctor?*, which was subtitled *Assessing quality of care in general practice*. This was the culmination of five years of labour by RCGP working parties. It recommended a form of evaluation which had been piloted by 35 assessment visits to practices in Merseyside and the south east of England. During these visits the assessors rated the GPs against a set of statements describing a 'model' practice. The statements (e.g. 'He [*sic*] can be seen quickly for urgent matters and normally within two days for non-urgent matters') were grouped into three areas: clinical competence, accessibility, and ability to communicate. It is striking how many basic features the RCGP scheme shares with CEPOD. It envisages an entirely voluntary process, based on peer review and oriented to professional education and development rather than any 'sharper' forms of remedial action. Like CEPOD it raises doubts about how far those doctors most in need of 'improvement' would be likely to volunteer for assessment, and like CEPOD it excludes the public – and management – from access to the judgements about the competence of individuals. Indeed:

> The second working party did in fact seriously consider soliciting the opinion of the practice's patients but concluded that this was not feasible. Furthermore, it would have detracted from the status of the assessment as a peer review (RCGP, 1985, p.7).

Soon after the RCGP's report, the government itself began to move on to the issue of standards in general practice. After a Green Paper and a period of consultation, the White Paper

Promoting Better Health: The government's programme for improving primary health care was published in November 1987 (DHSS et al, 1987). It dealt with a wide range of issues, at least four of which had direct bearing on the issues of quality, responsiveness and effectiveness. First, special pay incentives were proposed for GPs who offered certain preventive and educational services (for instance, reached certain targets for immunization and vaccination rates, and screening). These incentives were to be worked out through discussions with the profession. Second, incentives would also be introduced to raise general standards towards those obtaining in the best practices. Implementation of this general proposal would be worked out in consultation with the profession which had already shown considerable resistance to the idea of 'good practice allowances' (Davies, 1986). Subsequently, after some tortuous negotiations, GPs rejected the package and in mid-1989 the secretary of state imposed a new contract unilaterally. Third, FPCs would provide the public with more comprehensive information about practices, though this information appeared to be mainly descriptive of services provided and opening hours, rather than any direct measures of effectiveness or quality. Finally the complaints procedure was to be streamlined, and hearings were to be composed of equal numbers of professional and lay members. Clearly therefore, the DHSS/DoH acknowledged the accumulating evidence of considerable variance in the effectiveness, quality and responsiveness of GP services, and would like to do something about it. *Working for Patients* echoed *Promoting Better Health* in its determination to raise standards in general practice. As with hospital doctors, it proposed an extension of peer review and gave management (the FPCs) responsibility for seeing that this was put in place. Much will depend, however, on exactly what is worked out with the profession in respect both of peer review and of new incentive systems.

Managerial mechanisms

The mechanisms of Individual Performance Review (IPR) and Performance-Related Pay (PRP) were introduced during 1986 and were intended to apply to a new breed of post-Griffiths general managers at regional, district, unit and sub-unit levels. In a sense they were the final piece in the great new pyramid of objective-setting and monitoring that extended down from the ministerial reviews of regions. For now the *personal* objectives of individual managers could be explicitly defined, and aligned with the operational objectives of their unit/authority. According to the then chief executive of the NHS management board IPR 'establishes a direct link between corporate goals and those set for the individual' (Peach, 1988, p.43). Further, achievement of these personal objectives would be annually monitored, and additional pay awarded to those individuals who were adjudged to have performed particularly well. Beneath this surface impression of reasonableness and rationality, however, lurked a number of unanswered questions. Was the IPR system intended principally to monitor the short term performance of managers in carrying out plans, the personal development needs of those managers (as was sometimes stressed), the future promotability of the individual, or some combination of these, or something else altogether? What sort of issues would, in practice, come to dominate IPR agendas? How far would the IPR process, with its standardized forms and annual appraisal interviews, drift towards becoming a bureaucratic exercise, a process in which nothing really new was 'discovered', but the participants simply 'read off' obvious and largely achievable objectives from existing plans and commitments?

At the time of writing it is not yet possible to give definitive answers to these questions. Some tentative findings have, however, begun to emerge from the 1987–1989 Economic and Social Research Council research into the impact of general management (Harrison, Hunter, Marnoch and Pollitt, 1989a). It would appear that, for many UGMs and DGMs (though not all), IPR has been dominated by short-term targets for financial savings. There is also a tendency for a substantial proportion of the non-financial targets to be concerned with producing particular documents or setting up particular organizational arrangements by particular dates. In other words, apart from the achievement of financial targets, many of the objectives are actually of a rather 'introverted', process-oriented kind. What is more, there is something of a 'two-class society' among NHS managers, because many of the clinicians who have assumed general management posts do not take part in the IPR procedures, or, if they do, have much less to lose or gain from them than their non-clinician colleagues (since they are paid medical salaries and still have the security of their clinical posts to retreat to if their performance is judged unsatisfactory). Once more, therefore, it seems that a centrally-imposed monitoring scheme has been designed with economy and efficiency principally in mind, and that effectiveness, responsiveness and equity are not squarely addressed. Once more, also, the medical domain is largely immune from the monitoring process; IPRs are for *managers*, not for doctors other than for the small minority who 'wear two hats' by occupying management positions, at least on a short-term basis.

Public opinion

The 1980s not only witnessed an intensification of evaluatory activity by politicians, managers and the professions, but was also a period in which more and more sophisticated surveys of public opinion about the service were carried out. How did the consumers rate the NHS?

First, it has to be made clear that the surveys which have been mounted have varied widely in scope and intention. At one extreme, many health authorities have conducted small local surveys of groups of patients, sometimes with the intention of evaluating one quite narrow aspect of their services (hospital food for example), sometimes with broader intent (to collect patients' responses to entire episodes of treatment for example). Investigations of this kind may be very valuable to local management (or they may simply be filed away and ignored) but they are not pitched at the general level with which we are concerned, and nothing more will be said of them here.

At the other extreme, however, there have been a number of general, national surveys of public attitudes to the NHS (see, for example, Harrison, 1988a, pp.86–91 and Davies, 1989). There are at least five common denominators to their findings:

(1) Large majorities regularly express general satisfaction (or better) with the NHS (typically 70–80 per cent: see Davies, 1989).
(2) Among those who have recently received treatment, satisfaction levels tend to be even higher (typically 85–90 per cent)
(3) General practitioner services occasion less dissatisfaction than hospital services.
(4) This general satisfaction is unevenly distributed. The working class appears marginally less satisfied than the middle classes, men marginally less satisfied than women. Satisfaction also seems to increase with age, and the dissatisfaction of the young (under 24s) has been growing throughout the second half of the 1980s. There is also some regional variation, with London, the North West and Wales holding the lowest opinions of services in their areas.
(5) Substantial majorities indicate that they believe more should be spent on the NHS, and most of them would prefer this money to come from increased general taxation. Only about 10 per cent of the population appears to want to increase health care spending by having more private care,

and these 'privatizers' are disproportionately concentrated in Greater London, East Anglia and the South East.

In general terms, therefore (and bearing in mind the limitations of survey methodology) such public 'evaluations' usually come out strongly in favour of an NHS continuing along the present lines, funded rather more generously than hitherto, principally out of normal taxation. There is, however, some evidence of growing dissatisfaction, especially among the young and in particular parts of the country. Also, the questions posed in the surveys are seldom precise enough to allow us to distinguish between the different criteria (efficiency, effectiveness, responsiveness, equity) defined at the beginning of this chapter. Finally it should be pointed out that there is no guarantee that these public opinions would remain stable if larger numbers of people began to experience different kinds of service (e.g. through larger use of private facilities, or health services in other countries) and thus acquired some yardstick against which to compare the NHS.

Conceptual and technical difficulties

Since our dominant interest is in the way that power relationships have shaped the health policy process, it is possible that the discussion so far may have created the impression that the business of measuring the efficiency, effectiveness, responsiveness and equity of the NHS is actually relatively straightforward, and the sole reason for the still embryonic state of such measurement is the resistance of vested interests. If so, this would be misleading. There are genuine conceptual and technical difficulties involved in such measurement (Harrison and Long, 1989), and it is necessary to say something about these before proceeding to the final, interpretive section of this chapter.

The chief *conceptual* difficulties involved in evaluating health policies include the following:

1 Can we define 'health' in a way that commands common, or at least widespread support?
2 If we *can* thus define health, can we then proceed to define operational indicators of the presence or absence of 'health', preferably indicators which will show to what degree health is present ('health status') so that different states of healthiness/sickness can be compared?
3 If 1 and 2 can both be accomplished, do we then have theories available that will accurately tell us what changes in health

status will result from specified 'interventions' (e.g. providing a particular kind of health education programme, or screening service, or additional surgical service)?

If we can do all the foregoing, we may be in a position to act. But to choose the 'best' actions we will also need to have a set of values (about different health states) which will allow us to decide that ameliorating certain of these states is of higher priority than dealing with others. There will always be a need to prioritize because there will never be enough resources available to do everything that could, technically, be done for every person who could conceivably benefit from those interventions. Indeed, there is a cogent school of thought that suggests that, because of the rapid advance of medical technology, the gap between what we *could* do and what we can actually afford to do is widening all the time. Thus painful choices concerning what to 'leave out' are becoming more, not less, frequent. Arguably this would still be so even if we were able to eliminate all those procedures which are currently carried out but which are of little or no benefit to the patient.

Each of these conceptual 'requirements' is very taxing and, despite considerable scholarly and other efforts over the years, it is hard to think of many (if any) actual health programmes where even *one* of these requirements is fully satisfied. The philosophical difficulties associated with tackling such problems are large, and cannot be adequately summarized here (but see, for example Rivlin, 1971; March, 1978; Open University, 1988). In the space available we can probably do no more than indicate one major difficulty associated with each requirement.

Defining health in a way that commands general support has proved impossible. The most inclusive attempts seem to include virtually the whole of human life, while the more concrete and precise soon show themselves to be unhelpfully narrow or mechanistic. Probably the most famous effort was that of the World Health Organization, which concluded that health consisted of a 'state of complete physical, mental and social wellbeing, not merely the absence of disease and infirmity'. On this view few policies and few agencies would *not* be health policies or health agencies – health would expand beyond all manageable bounds (though some would say that that is precisely what is needed). This kind of definition is often contrasted with much narrower 'scientific' definitions of disease as negative health, which are usually derived from the medical model developed in Western societies during the nineteenth century. The rise of this set of beliefs was associated with the growing authority of the medical profession (Allsop, 1984, ch.8). Thus you may feel ill, but you are not officially suffering from a disease – and thereby entitled to treatment – until a qualified medical practitioner says you are. Medical definitions tend to exclude or downgrade a number of subjectives states ('depression' for example) and to result in agencies and policies devoted to eliminating medically-defined disease rather than promoting more broadly – and possibly subjectively – defined good health.

It will already be apparent how hard it will be to define good operational indicators of health status. In so far as definitions of health include some subjective elements (how the sick individual *feels*; what the degree of distress or discomfort is) they necessarily import large problems of interpersonal comparisons. Thus, if I say that I feel great discomfort, how can we be sure that this is equivalent to anyone else saying they feel great discomfort? Even more objective indicators are frequently hard to interpret. Take the example of hospital waiting lists, which figured prominently in the debates of the mid and late 1980s concerning the extent to which the NHS was failing to meet the community's needs. If a particular waiting list went down this was usually greeted as a success, a cause for congratulation. But were waiting lists actually a good indicator of the success of the hospital services in meeting needs? A falling list could be due to increased surgical productivity – an efficiency gain by which the same number of surgeons, nurses and paramedics were now able to get through more operations of a given type per year than formerly. Unfortunately, however, this was not the only possible or legitimate interpretation. The same fall could be due to administrators going through an old list simply weeding out the names of those patients who had died or moved to another area or had the operation done privately. (Shortening lists in this way was actually quite a popular exercise at the time of writing.) Or the fall could result from local GPs despairing of the very long list and cutting back on the number of their patients they referred to the hospital in question. Or the productivity gain could have been real, but achieved only by moving resources out of some other area of the hospital, where patients were now paying, in one way or another, for the better prospects of their fellow citizens on the surgery waiting list. Finally, the fall in the waiting list could have been real and accomplished without depleting other areas, yet it might have been achieved at the cost of lower quality – more unsuccessful operations, more early readmissions, perioperative deaths and so on. The waiting list statistics alone would not tell us which of these very different processes, or which combination of them, lay behind the apparently laudable reduction. The third major conceptual difficulty in the evaluation of health care services is the frequent inadequacy of the action theories available to policy makers when they are called upon to respond to perceived problems. Even when a clear definition of health has been established, and valid and reliable indicators of the presence or absence of health are to hand, is there anything of *known* effectiveness which can be done? Many medical authorities suggest that reliable and effective interventions are rarer than most patients (and politicians) would like to think (Cochrane, 1972; McKeown, 1980). One commentator explains:

> A few patients will always be cured whatever treatment is used because of the placebo effect. Since doctors and patients tend to be optimists, a successful recovery will usually be attributed to the particular treatment or management the patient was given. Doctors may then repeat that form of treatment on future occasions without considering whether it is appropriate (Holland, 1983, p.xiv).

The requisite action theories would have to include not merely specified medical interventions, of proven effectiveness, but also designs for the optimal organizational arrangements to carry these medical procedures to the needy populace. It will be glaringly apparent to those who have read the previous chapters of this book that there are as yet few settled and uncontested organizational forms in the field of health care. The worldwide debate over how to organize to combat AIDS is simply the latest and most dramatic example of the continuing arguments about the relative effectiveness and efficiency of hospital versus community-based forms of care, medical versus paramedical versus lay therapies, large centralized institutions versus small, local institutions, and so on.

The final conceptual problem is perhaps the most intractable of all. One can only evaluate a policy against a set of objectives. A prerequisite for a stable set of objectives is an underlying, equally stable, set of priorities and, underpinning that, a clear set of values. In the real world of British health care politics, however, it is far from certain whether any such sturdy pyramid of values, priorities and objectives has ever existed. Some public sympathies (e.g. for small children with life-threatening diseases, or for mothers-to-be) appear fairly constant, but these hardly amount to a comprehensive listing of all the health states which health service staff and health care policymakers have to deal with. *Comparison* seems to be one of the most awkward and most avoided issues. As we saw in Chapter 3, the elderly, the mentally ill and the mentally handicapped are designated priority groups, but – in a world of little or no growth in real resources per capita – who should be put in the less-than-priority category? Conceptually and morally, how can decisions like this be formulated and, eventually, taken? Politicians and managers alike have shown little enthusiasm for tackling these questions, yet broad evaluation of health policies (as opposed to the narrower evaluation of specific therapies or organizational arrangements) is – strictly – impossible without a set of priorities as a yardstick. The present situation is one in which actual priorities seem to emerge from:

> Complete and largely unco-ordinated clinical freedom, coupled with the politics of the ballot box and pressure group (letters, demonstrations and various other forms of 'shroud waving', accompanied by lotteries and collection tins) (Open University, 1988, Introtext 08, p.13).

However, it has to be said that even if some statespersonlike leader, or party, were prepared to take on the thankless task of exposing to the mass public the nature and consequences of prioritization (i.e. rationing) in health care (at *any* given level of resources) there would be no guarantee of an illuminating outcome. There can be no a *priori* assumption that any active consensus exists (or could be assembled) concerning the operational priorities which should be pursued by the NHS (Mulkay *et al*, 1987). Furthermore, even if such a consensus could, slowly and painfully, be assembled, what chance would it have of surviving over the kind of time periods necessary for planning major changes in the pattern of health services? So many influences could begin to shift public opinion – the development of dramatic new medical technologies; the occurrence of 'scandals' such as those which fuelled the policy priority given to reforming long-stay institutions in the late 1960s and early 1970s; the appearance of new diseases (like AIDS); or ideological shifts in the perceived 'worth' of certain groups in society (e.g. the elderly, drug abusers).

This has been an exceedingly brief inspection of some of the conceptual problems standing in the way of an evaluation of health care services and policies. To these must be added more *technical* difficulties, which would still have to be surmounted even if the conceptual problems could be resolved. Again, only a summary indication of the nature of these difficulties can be afforded. They fall mainly under the headings of time, cost and complexity.

As far as time is concerned, two major issues are the timeliness of the available data and the appropriate timescale for evaluation. The collection, storage and collation of data on a population of fifty-five million was for a long time an enormous and time-consuming manual task. The result was often that national or regional data only appeared long after their immediate relevance to operational management – or even policymaking – was on the wain. The rapid spread of computerized record keeping should – in principle – significantly shrink this problem, *if* the very complex problems of harmonizing different computer systems operated by different agencies can be resolved.

Timescale difficulties are less tractable. Some diseases, and some consequences (side effects) of medical interventions, take very long periods of time to manifest themselves. Some of the cancers allegedly induced by working at the Windscale/Sellafield nuclear reprocessing plant may not appear for twenty or thirty years after the initial exposure, often after the worker concerned has retired or moved to another job. Health education programmes designed to change behaviour in respect of, say, eating or drinking habits may not impact fully on mortality or mobidity indicators for similarly long periods. The evaluation of these processes can therefore only take place over timescales much longer than those in which politicians and managers are usually interested.

Cost is another problem, probably a more pervasive one than time. All monitoring requires some resources. So to monitor and evaluate is, in effect, to divert some resources (money, staff, time) out of immediate patient care. Looked at in this way it can be appreciated that, good though it may be to evaluate, this good always has to be traded off against the benefits that might have flowed from other possible applications of the resources so used. That is, evaluation has an opportunity cost, it is not a free good. This principle was clearly illustrated in the late 1980s when a number of health authorities found it a slow struggle to implement the new information systems recommended by the Korner reports, not because the new systems were not useful but rather because of the difficulties of diverting the necessary resources. There is thus a question of *how much* evaluation is optimal, and this has both technical and conceptual aspects.

Finally, it is hard to overestimate the sheer complexity of the data collection systems that would ideally be required to generate reliable and timely data about the efficiency, effectiveness, responsiveness and equity of health care services. Individual patients would need to be followed from their GPs, through outpatient and inpatient episodes and then back into their homes. Records would also need to be 'portable' between local authority services, FPCs, health authorities and private health care agencies.

Only a set of such cumulative records would fully reveal the patterns of usage of different groups of health care consumers, and show which patterns tended to produce the most effective, efficient (etc.) outcomes. Even these would ideally need to be supplemented by the inclusion of other highly health-relevent information, such as significant changes in the individual's diet, pattern of exercise, working conditions, lifestyle, and so on. Needless to say, actual and currently planned record systems conspicuously lack this comprehensiveness. On the contrary, they are heavily structured by existing divisions between different parts of the health service and social services, and between public and private sectors.

Interpretation

That the conceptual and technical difficulties of evaluating health services and policies are so formidable should not blind us to the more 'political' factors discussed earlier in the chapter. For, difficult though evaluation may be, there remains a clear pattern in *what* has been attempted, and by *whom*. The dominant concerns in the 1950s, and again in the 1980s, have been economy and efficiency. The chief 'bearers' of this concern have been government, Parliament and, more recently, managers within health authorities. Effectiveness and clinical quality, in so far as they have been tackled at all, have been entrusted almost exclusively to the medical profession. The (few) attempts to assess effectiveness by other groups (for example the College of Health's guide to hospital waiting lists) have been attacked by the medical profession, and have received little support from government. The main exceptions to these generalizations have, notably, occurred in those parts of the health service where doctors are not as numerous or dominant as they usually are in hospitals: 'The field of preventive health care has been subjected to particularly thorough evaluation when compared to curative or caring services' (Holland, 1983, p.xiv). Holland suggests that this difference is due to the fact that 'Those involved in planning preventive programmes are frequently more numerate than clinicians or come from the numerate scientific disciplines. They may therefore be more interested in evaluation'. This kind of explanation may be accurate as far as it goes, but does not address the deeper question of why clinicians have continued to be able to resist any pressures to become more numerate, 'scientific', and self-evaluative. The traditional medical education has remained stubbornly individualistic, and has emphasized the uniqueness of the doctor–patient relationship rather than the analysis of community health needs.

In explaining why so little *attempt* has been made to tackle some types of evaluation, some of our four theories of the distribution of power seem to perform better than others. All have some explanatory power, but public choice approaches and neo-pluralist theories appear to have some fairly obvious limitations.

First, let us take public choice theories. In so far as these place great emphasis on *ownership status* (public versus private ownership of health care providing agencies), they are somewhat unconvincing. As the authors of an ESRC research project into organizational performance explain:

> Public choice theory is strong on *a priori* reasoning but short on empiricism. Studies undertaken into public versus private efficiency in a number of countries suggest that market competition is more important than ownership in determining performance (Dunsire *et al*, 1988).

In other words, a private hospital is not likely to be more efficient than a public hospital but a hospital which has to compete with another hospital (whether either or both are public or private) is likely to be more efficient than the one which does not. The focus should therefore be on competition rather than on simple public/private dichotomies in ownership status, and, to be fair, this is where some of the more careful public choice theorists put it. (See, for instance Peet, 1987.)

Unfortunately, this still does not take us very far in understanding the development of evaluation in British health care. The public choice focus is quite narrow. Efficiency is the overwhelming concern: so much so that, in one well-publicized recent study, other performance criteria were relegated to a single, unsubstantiated sentence:

> As for commercialism threatening standards, no better way has yet been found of judging the extent to which they are met than through open competition – with loss of client or contract the result of not measuring up (Peet, 1987, p.8).

This statement simply ignores the massive international literature documenting how very difficult it frequently is for health care consumers to make rational judgements about standards, if the latter are taken to mean effectiveness and quality. It also overlooks mounting evidence that standards may indeed be at risk where a competitive climate prevails. For example, early in 1988 a

London FPC withdrew consent for its sixty GPs to use a particular commercial deputizing service because of concern about an 'unsatisfactory' standard of service. Yet this deputizing service operated in the capital, where at least a dozen other commercial competitors might have been expected, according to public choice theory, to ensure high standards (Feinmann, 1988).

So even in relation to the efficiency criterion, public choice theory is not always a clear or reliable guide. Why, if a public monopoly supplier is so immune to efficiency considerations, have economy and efficiency actually been a continuing concern of governments and a focus for much more governmentally-driven activity than effectiveness or responsiveness? This does not sound like the predicted collusion between budget-maximizing DHSS/DoH civil servants and budget and status-maximizing consultants and hospital administrations, at least not during the efficiency-conscious 1980s. On the contrary, the story is one of increasing tension and conflict between the DHSS and health authorities, culminating in a major, media-drenched 'crisis' in the latter part of 1987. Also, how does public choice theory explain the more substantial history of evaluation in preventive, public health than in the hospitals? Here is an area with virtually no competition at all – at the heart of the public sector – yet evaluation is evidently more active and open than elsewhere.

Another weakness in the public choice approach is its extreme, and sometimes virtually unargued, scepticism concerning the scope for administrative and organizational reform (*unless* this is tied to the forces of the market). It is a perspective which would have little to say about initiatives such as the review process or PIs. Typical is Peet's dismissal:

> The bureaucrat's way is to commission endless audits and press for better management practices (1987, p.7).

This line of argument not merely understates the potential significance (and complexity) of organizational reform, it also fails to explain why, for example, administrative costs in the predominantly private, competitive US health care system represent approximately two and a half times the percentage of total costs which they do in the supposedly more 'bureaucratic' British system.

In sum, the public choice perspective is a narrow one, concentrating on the efficiency criterion and usually having rather little to say about effectiveness or equity. Even so on its own ground (efficiency) it often exhibits an *a priori* overconfidence about the powers of competition to ensure *both* greater efficiency *and* the maintenance of quality. Correspondingly, it has little to say about the kind of managerial and organizational changes which have made up a good part of the thin history of evaluation within the NHS, or about contrasts between different parts of the health services. Perhaps it is at its strongest in focusing on the professional monopoly possessed by doctors as a likely barrier to the evaluation of performance.

Neo-pluralism does not seem to be an overwhelmingly helpful perspective either. In practice, for most of the life of the NHS there has not been a vigorous debate between different groups concerning the performance of the NHS and how it might be evaluated. Even central government did not begin to take a very active role until the late 1970s, and then it confined itself largely to matters of economy and efficiency. Nor was there any sustained pressure from the medical profession – or any of the other major provider groups – to establish better measures of need or equity. Most tellingly (for the pluralist image of a fairly open, bargained group process) such debates as there have been about evaluation seem to have been among a very restricted set of participants and have only very occasionally and briefly exercised Parliament or the political parties. The consumer lobby, though potentially vast, has been conspicuously unable to 'punch its weight', and has seldom gained the access to the government's inner councils which the medical profession has been able to enjoy as a matter of course. Nor is the notion of bargaining a particularly accurate characterization of what has often happened. Ministerial reviews, PIs and the HAS were all introduced rather quickly, in response to salient political embarrassments. They were not the outcomes of long processes of consultation, still less bargaining.

The neo-pluralist perspective is perhaps more useful in relation to what not to expect. Thus it has certainly been the case that policy monitoring has been handicapped by the continuing absence of any clear statement of the NHS's priorities. Here the model of a plurality of competing interests does help us to understand why it is politically uncomfortable to have well-defined objectives. Similarly, the neo-pluralist emphasis on the privileged position of big business throws light on the discreet, off-stage way in which the DHSS's relationships with the multinational pharmaceutical companies have usually been conducted. No drama or governmental accusations here. Nor, until the early 1980s, was there much government action to tackle the recurring problem of substantial cost overruns during the construction, by private construction companies, of major new hospitals. Finally, despite all the recent tightening up in the monitoring of efficiency in NHS hospitals, the DHSS/DoH has been noticably slow to tackle the issues of efficiency and quality in private health care services (Higgins, 1983; Feinmann, 1988).

Our remaining two perspectives – neo-élitist and neo-Marxist – seem to explain the history of evaluation rather more fully (scope), and with fewer (though still some) inconsistencies with the evidence. They are to some extent complementary to each other, élitism providing a good explanation of the foreground (institutional level) of our 'pocket history', while Marxism helps in explaining how that foreground might be connected to the larger social framework.

The élitists' model of a powerful medical profession goes a long way towards explaining why the monitoring of effectiveness has moved so slowly in both public and private sectors. Of course, the greater cost and conceptual difficulties of effectivenes-monitoring have provided convenient rationalizations for constantly postponing (as in the PI exercise) major initiatives on this front. Efficiency, on the other hand, can be measured 'in house' (inputs and outputs). Notice, also that the cautious start that is at last being made on effectiveness monitoring is still largely the 'private property' of the profession (CEPOD and negotiations over good practice allowances in primary care). Even the 1989 White Paper is insistent that 'Medical audit is essentially a professional matter' (Department of Health *et al*, 1989b, p.39). Consumer organizations – or even other provider groups such as the nurses or paramedics – are not welcome round these negotiating tables. Unlike the medical profession these other groups cannot offer the government the exchange benefits both of disciplining their members *and* of carrying the responsibility for dispersing, legitimating (and largely concealing) the politically poisonous rationing decisions (Harrison, 1988a, p.125) as to which would-be consumers get what, and in what order of priority. To the élitist the implicit 'deal' would seem to have been that as long as the medical profession continued to perform both these functions tolerably well, government, for its part, would not seek to insist on tight monitoring of effectiveness, efficiency or responsiveness. Of course, other provider groups do to some extent discipline their members (especially, perhaps, the Royal College of Nursing, favoured by the prime minister in the 'crisis' of 1988 because of their acceptance of a no-strike clause). But their work roles are often defined *in relation to* the much more dominant doctors. And, crucially, they have nothing like the same influence as the doctors in respect of the *de facto* rationing of health services. Thus the role of the medical profession's 'peak associations' in relation to government has a higher 'intermediation' component than is present for most other provider groups (Crouch, 1983).

This close and mediating relationship between government and the medical profession helps explain a number of the details of the evidence reviewed in this chapter. Thus even the efficiency drives such as Rayner scrutinies and cost improvement programmes have been targeted mainly on support, paramedical and nursing services, not on the clinical heartland; likewise the new 'consumerist' initiatives aimed at improving the Service's responsiveness (Harrison, Hunter, Marnoch and Pollitt, 1989a). Similarly, if we enquire where some progress has been made in respect of quality and effectiveness, we find it has been in areas where doctors are either thin on the ground (preventive health services), belong to lower status specialisms ('cinderella services' – HAS), or both. Thus, if the kind of crisis over funding and priorities which blew up at the end of 1987 were to continue, the benefits of medical autonomy for the government might not appear quite so substantial. The close controls proposed in the 1989 White Paper – medical audit, resource management, indicative drug budgets for GPs and tighter job definitions for consultants – may reflect precisely this kind of government exasperation.

The neo-Marxist perspective complements the élitist account by reminding us that any 'bargain' is struck within a particular socio-economic context, and that changes in the context may render the bargain less attractive to one or both parties. If, in the 1990s, capitalism is in crisis and the accumulation process requires radical reductions in 'social consumption expenditure' coupled with the privatization of extensive public assets (see, for example, Navarro, 1984) then this may ultimately oblige government to tackle medical autonomy. After cost-improvement programmes have squeezed savings out of non-clinical areas, and competitive tendering has 'privatized' many 'hotel' and support services, the pressure for 'rationalization' may have to be turned directly onto the citadel of clinical freedom. Part of such a campaign would have to be the production of quantitative measures of some kind that would legitimate the sought-after interventions. An exposure of widespread inefficiencies or widely varying standards of care would serve as just such a justification. Under such circumstances one might expect hostilities to begin to disfigure a formerly discreet and cosy relationship, and the government to attempt to exploit internal divisions within the medical profession, rewarding those doctors who acknowledged the need for rationalization and freezing out the others. Here one can see the characteristic conflict-focus of the Marxist model. Doctors might be part of the bourgeoisie, but if economies are in crisis, some of them at least may have to be sacrificed in favour of sustaining the rate of profit and the collective security of the capitalist classes.

Much hangs, of course, on the identification of 'crisis'. Is there one, and if so, what is its nature? The Marxist record of prediction in these matters has been, to say the least, disappointing. On the other hand, there *does* seem to have been an inverse relationship between economic growth and the pressure central government has put on the NHS to improve its efficiency. The long boom from the mid-1950s to the mid-1970s witnessed much less activity on this front than the more economically troubled periods before (Guillebaud) and since. There is also a problem with some Marxist accounts of the role of the NHS. If it is meant to be functionally useful in maintaining the health of the labour force, why have its wards and waiting rooms always been full of the elderly and children? If, on the other hand, its main function has been to legitimate government and symbolize a unified public interest, then why has Mrs Thatcher concluded that the late 1980s – a time when the economy is claimed to be rather more robust than for a while – is an appropriate time to destabilize the structures of 1948 and 1972 and begin to encourage private forms of care?

These considerations take us some way from our main focus on the history of monitoring and evaluation – and that itself is quite characteristic of a broad structural approach such as Marxism. Perhaps its main strength is to remind us that there are powerful structural reasons why, in a capitalist state, government monitoring of a tax-financed health service is always likely to be first and foremost directed at holding down expenditures. Marxists, also, would be thoroughly unsurprised that government and professional interest in assessing how far the NHS has provided a truly equitable set of services has been fitful and lukewarm. A capitalist state, on this analysis, will be quite willing to claim credit for an institution which symbolizes 'care for all the nation', but will be simultaneously reluctant to investigate what actually happens at the grass roots, knowing that the resulting empirical data would almost certainly highlight the gross inequalities of social class which actually characterize the deep structure of capitalist society. To some extent these insights possess an explanatory value independently of whether the larger claims that some Marxists make concerning crises can be sustained or not.

Concluding reflections

The neo-Marxist and neo-élitist perspectives thus seem particularly valuable in explaining the broad evolution of evaluation within the NHS. Nevertheless, their usefulness has its limits.

They are at their most useful at the level at which this chapter has been pitched: that of general national or system-wide developments. These theories, perhaps neo-Marxism especially, are less valuable in explaining regional or local variations. Why, for example, have the surgeons of Lothian been running a system of surgical audit for more than a decade? Why do neurological traumas in Glasgow or bowel cancers in London attract intensive intra-professional evaluation while many other conditions – or the same conditions in other places – do not? (Devlin, 1988, pp.306–9). Why has Scotland been six years behind England and Wales in developing performance indicators, and why has it adopted a review process which is substantially different from its counterpart south of the border?

We cannot provide detailed answers to these questions here. In general terms, however, explanation of such phenomena would seem to require a closer study of local élite networks, local institutional variations and differences in local political and resource climates. In Scotland, for example, aggregate resource levels have been higher than in England (Chapter 3) and the one-tier connections between Health Boards and the SHHD have been more intimate than is possible in the larger, two-tiered English system. Such features may offer local élites opportunities to get things done (and other things delayed or stopped) which make that country (or health authority or medical specialism) 'unusual'. Variations of these kinds are interesting in that they frequently undermine what were articles of faith elsewhere in the system. Thus (to take one further example) all those English consultants who, in the late 1980s, vehemently opposed the suggestion that their contracts might be held by the authority in which they worked (rather than by the RHA) presumably ignored the situation in Wales, where their colleagues appeared to manage perfectly well with exactly the arrangement so feared in England.

One final reflection is that this is a particularly exciting time to be studying the measurement and evaluation of health care. After more than three decades of little movement (apart from local or particular initiatives of the kind referred to above) evaluation has now moved squarely onto the national political agenda. As one consultant surgeon recently put it:

The concept of medical quality as the exclusive preserve of doctors can no longer be maintained. Computers and consumerism have allowed others to invade our turf . . . Every one of us, doctors and patients, is inextricably caught up in today's political and philosophical whirlwind. Advancing technology, expanding expectations, and escalating public expenditure dictate that change must occur (Devlin, 1988, p.317).

This part, at least, of the settlement of 1946–8 is now under renegotiation. It remains to be seen where, in the three-cornered space between doctors, managers and consumers, the new deal will be struck. Neither of the two theories which have proved most useful in explaining the past would lead us to be particularly optimistic for the empowerment of consumers. The contest seems more likely to take place principally between managers, increasingly the bearers of the concerns of government, and doctors, defending their autonomy.

6 The dynamics of health policy

Our main purpose in writing this book is to identify and analyse the main forces shaping UK health policy since the early 1970s, though we hope and expect that the material presented in Chapters 2 to 4 and the Annexe has served the secondary purpose of informing the reader about the content of that policy and about the institutions of the NHS. It is now time to concentrate on that primary task and to draw together the threads of our analysis.

One thing which should be immediately evident to the reader is how little change of any substance (other than in overall funding) has been wrought, until recently, by those ostensibly in charge of the Service: the policymakers in government and the NHS's managers. This observation, as far as it goes, is not inconsistent with the 'shared version' of events in the health sector in the 1960s and 1970s which we outlined in Chapter 1. But we need to beware of the assumption that particular theoretical approaches are appropriate simply because we find some points of congruence.

We commence our concluding analysis, therefore, by arguing, that, despite some consonances, the 'shared version' is not sufficiently consistent with the events of the last decade to constitute an adequate explanation; indeed, as we hinted in Chapter 1, it is somewhat less than adequate even in respect of the earlier period. We also wish to argue that neither neo-pluralist nor public choice theories will suffice for our purposes, and devote a section to re-visiting each of these in the light of our descriptive material from Chapters 2 to 5. Our own attempt at an adequate explanation is based on combining and modifying neo-élite and neo-Marxist theories; we discuss each of these separately before relating them to each other. Our final section examines the implications of our analysis for the future of the NHS.

The shared version re-visited

In Chapter 1 we had a good deal to say about what we regarded as the lack of *comprehensiveness* and *coherence* of the shared version. We also hinted that we did not regard it as *consistent* with much of the evidence in Chapters 2 to 5. Let us summarize some of these inconsistencies.

First, PMA: it is clear from our accounts of the poor implementation of priorities, the behaviour of managers (Chapter 3), the pattern of 'managerial relations' and the ability of local consultants to frustrate national agreements (Chapter 4), and the ability of doctors to keep evaluation of their activities optional and within the profession (Chapter 5), that at local level, and on a wide range of issues, there simply are no partisans. Doctors dominate. It should also be noted that, while the issues that we have chosen to examine in this book do tend to support the 'shared version's' contention that medical power is mainly defensive, there is evidence that on other issues, especially innovation in medicine, medical influence can be pro-active too (Stocking, 1985, pp.30–46).

Second, incremental analysis: while we concede that this is a good description of managerial behaviour, at least until recently, it should be evident to the reader that this has certainly not been the case at government levels, where some rather radical policies have been devised. Examples include the RAWP formula for the redistribution of finance, the introduction of health care priorities outside acute medicine, the replacement of consensus decision-making by general managers, and recent proposals for internal competition (see Chapter 3.) The fact that the actual results of implementing these policies have often been modest (incremental *politics*) does not result from incremental *analysis*.

Finally, political consensus; this is a difficult topic, since it is never clear at one particular time to what extent apparent lack of consensus is merely rhetorical. Thus, Labour Party opposition to Griffiths and *Working for Patients* may not be a reliable indicator of what might occur if there were to be a change of government. (We return to this below.) But even at the level of rhetoric, if such it is, the contrast between current controversy and the consensus over the introduction of the 1974 Reorganization of the NHS (Harrison, 1988a, pp.15–17) is marked. Moreover, *Working for Patients* clearly challenges what we described earlier as the *internal* political consensus; by threatening greater managerial control over doctors, it moves away from the implicit bargain of 1946–8.

Neo-pluralist theory re-visited

Our descriptions of health policies in the preceding chapters display some obvious points of fit with neo-pluralist theory. Two aspects of these events offer themselves as tempting candidates, though on closer examination neither turns out to bear such analysis.

First, there has been a reasonable amount of pressure group activity in several of our policy areas. In Chapter 3 we noted CBI lobbying (note the involvement of big business) about the size of the NHS workforce (see also Harrison, 1988a, pp.98–9), and lobbying by pressure groups representing clients such as the elderly and mentally ill. In Chapter 4 we noted the increasing intensity of trade union activity in the 1970s, and saw how pressure from junior doctors' representatives helped to keep the issue of medical careers on the government agenda. But, crucially, in none of these cases was such lobbying decisive in producing the eventual outcome of policies, even if it did influence their formal content. And in Chapter 5 we saw that there has been no substantial debate about performance evaluation, perhaps the single area where one would most expect to see lobbying by interested parties.

Second, Parliament (in practice, the House of Commons Select Committees) has had an important role since 1981 in focusing the attention of the government on NHS performance (see Chapters 3 and 5), an activity which has triggered some organizational changes that would otherwise probably not have occurred. But Parliament did not determine the form of such change, which (as is shown in some detail in Harrison, 1988a, ch.6) more than once resulted from unexpected proposals.

On closer examination, therefore, neo-pluralist theory looks less attractive, and even less so if we examine the role of the state (a central element in neo-pluralist analysis) in our policy areas. In none of these do we see the government occupying the role of ostensible referee between competing interests, occasionally intervening to tip the balance on issues vital to itself. In the event, the government has performed two different roles, on different issues, neither corresponding to that postulated in neo-pluralist analysis. On three policy areas, funding of the NHS, market relations with staff, and the form of organization, the government's role has been decisive. On our remaining four topics, priority groups, resource allocation, managerial relations with staff (in which we include the medical careers topic), and evaluation, the government has produced policies, sometimes in response to lobbying, but, as we have seen, none of these has so far been decisive in producing their *ostensible* desired outcome. (We emphasize 'ostensible' because it highlights a point to which we return in our penultimate section.)

Public choice theory re-visited

Unlike the case of neo-pluralist theory, we cannot say that there is very much consistency at all between the material that we set out in Chapters 2 to 5 and public choice theory. It will be recalled that the latter starts from the notion of public sector bureaucrats pursuing their own interests by 'empire building', with a resulting oversupply of the services provided by their organizations. Although we did observe such personal welfare maximization in Chapter 4, it was on the part of doctors, and did not really take the form of empire building, but rather of protecting the quality of working life. This is not, of course, to say that NHS managers never attempt to pursue their own interests; the formal organization of the NHS has often been partly the product of occupational politics (Harrison, 1988a, pp.27–8), and certainly the administrators were swift to seize the opportunity to turn themselves into general managers offered by the 1983 Griffiths Report (Social Services Committee, 1984; Harrison, 1988a, table 4.1). But these observations do not explain the events which we have described in the preceding chapters.

Indeed, far from an oversupply of health care having occurred, funding has been quite tightly restricted in recent years, as Chapter 2 has noted; in this respect, new right theorists such as Seldon (1980) who have written specifically about health services (rather than, as Niskanen did, about the public sector in general) are right to say that, without an NHS, a greater proportion of the gross domestic product would be devoted to health care. As we noted in Chapter 1, different new right theories contradict each other. Yet the remarkable thing is that the theories propose the same solution for their contradictory versions of the problem; the application of market principles.

Here we can, of course, see a link with some of our descriptive material; the proposals in the White Paper *Working for Patients* (see Annexe) are very much cast in this mould, though, as we noted in Chapter 5, *strictly* speaking, a public choice theorist would insist on a change of ownership, rather than just internal competition. Does this, then, provide in some sense an explanation of at least one event in our account of health policy? Can we simply say that the *Working for Patients* proposals represent the ideology of a new right Conservative government? While at one level this is self-evidently true (though the government's conversion to such a view would have to be relatively recent, as is clear from Chapter 3), there is no obvious link between party ideology and the rest of our descriptive material: no obvious link with funding or pay settlements, for instance – precisely the issues on which one would expect party ideology to count, if it counts at all.

Moreover, current international interest in internal markets in health care goes well beyond Conservative politicians and includes at least one socialist government in Europe (personal communication). We prefer, therefore, to adopt Klein's (1984) view of ideology as something which is used to provide a *post facto* rationalization of action already decided upon, and to seek a more *comprehensive* theoretical explanation of the dynamics of British health policy.

Neo-élite theory re-visited

As we saw in Chapter 1, neo-élite theory is often concerned with occupational élites, and our descriptive chapters have shown the effectiveness of one group of doctors, hospital consultants, in obstructing the implementation of national priorities in health care and resource allocation (Chapter 3), in evading managerial control (Chapter 4), and in avoiding a potentially threatening debate about the evaluation of services (Chapter 5). Change in these areas has been, at best, incremental (incremental *politics*). But this, largely defensive, influence has not been exerted in open conflict with governments. Rather, it has been achieved through a monopoly of *local* legitimacy, which has tended to prevent managers from seriously attempting to implement national policies, even where these (as in the case of the consultant:junior ratio) have been agreed at national level with the profession itself. National policies have, in a real sense, been kept off the effective local agenda, an exercise in what in Chapter 1 we referred to as the 'second face' of power (Bachrach and Baratz, 1970).

Nevertheless, two problems remain to be overcome before we can be confident about the usefulness of neo-élite theory. Firstly, although its scope (comprehensiveness) is quite wide, there is a significant proportion of our descriptive material which it does not explain; three of our policy areas, funding (Chapter 2), organization structure (Chapter 3) and market relations (Chapter 4) were not dominated by the medical profession, but by the government. We shall return to this in the following two sections.

Second, no single one of the neo-élite theories that we summarized in Chapter 1 is consistent with the whole of the period covered by our descriptive material. Liberal corporatism, despite first appearances and the assertions of writers such as Cawson (1982), is not consistent with events. As already noted in Chapter 4, up to about 1981, there was little or no managerial challenge to the consultant dominance, and (following Dunleavy,

1981) we characterized this as 'ideological corporatism', to signify the medical monopoly of legitimacy. But from 1982, and more especially after the introduction in 1984 of general management, there has been a managerial challenge to this legitimacy, even though (as Chapter 4 shows) this has certainly not so far had the effect of subordinating doctors to managers. As we note in Chapters 3 and 4 and the Annexe, the *Working for Patients* proposals are likely to add impetus to this challenge. From this time onwards, therefore, the Dunleavy model cannot be regarded as appropriate.

More appropriate subsequently is Alford's (1975) model of structural interests in which a dominant interest – in our case, as in Alford's own case study of New York – the medical 'professional monopolists', exists alongside a challenging interest – in our and cases as Alford's – the management 'corporate rationalizers', who seek to obtain managerial control over the professionals. Our emphasis here is somewhat different from that of some exponents of the 'shared version' (see, for instance, Heller, 1979; Allsop, 1984; Ham, 1985). Although we agree with these authors that an underlying theme of successive NHS reorganizations has been a higher managerial and financial profile, of which doctors have certainly been aware, we depart from the 'shared version' in our judgement that it is only during the 1980s that the challenge to doctors has acquired substance. It is now more focused and more confrontational; whereas earlier managerial developments stressed consensus and collegiate relationships, the stress now is on incentives for behavioural change.

We suggest that, until the watershed of the early 1980s, and despite the 1974 reforms, managers were more often facilitators, even allies of the dominant medical interest. The challenge to doctors lay primarily in the realm of philosophies (such as integration), or at the micro level in exploiting competing subdivisions within the profession in order to resolve issues of local resource allocation. In our judgement, these did not amount to anything like the broad-scope assertion of managerial prerogatives which has begun to emerge in the 1980s. This is not the same thing as saying that managers have actually become more powerful than doctors; Alford's theory does not predict the outcome of the challenge, which remains to be discovered empirically. As we noted in Chapter 4, post-Griffiths research does not so far indicate major changes in managerial–medical power relationships. But the ostensible challenge of internal markets suggests that post-White Paper relationships will be a fruitful topic for research.

What is needed, therefore, is some way, not inconsistent with élite theory, in which we can explain both the policies (funding, organization structure and market relations) which neo-élite theory does not, and the transition during 1981 to 1984 from a situation with a single, medical, elite to two competing élites. Can we combine theories so as to provide comprehensive, coherence, and consistency with our descriptive material? We shall attempt to do this in our penultimate section. But first we must re-visit neo-Marxist theory.

Neo-Marxist theory re-visited

We saw in Chapter 1 that élites are important for neo-Marxists too, but that the interest of such theorists lies in relating élites to the class structure of the capitalist state. This interest is not merely a scholastic concern with the categorization of particular occupations into social classes but rather an attempt to investigate the function of élites in supporting or challenging the capitalist state. Our analysis so far has emphasized the influence of the medical profession as an élite, and we have noted that most doctors are employed in the NHS. It is likely, therefore, that in neo-Marxist analysis the function of the profession will be closely linked to the function of the welfare state, and the NHS in particular. It will be readily apparent from what we said in Chapter 1 that, in neo-Marxist terms, the NHS can be regarded as constituting both 'social investment' and 'social expenses'; that is, it helps to maintain a healthy workforce and to legitimate the capitalist system.

Several neo-Marxist writers (such as O'Connor, 1973 and Offe, 1984) have posited an eventual 'crisis of the welfare state'; at some risk of oversimplification (and there are differences between individual writers), the argument runs as follows. Demand for welfare state expenditure rises over time, as a result of a number of factors; demographic changes and public expectations are amongst those frequently cited. At some point, however, capitalists begin to resist this trend, calculating that the resulting increases in taxation will erode profitability, and that the public services are bidding too strongly for labour, perhaps bidding up wage levels in the process. The government cannot easily respond to these concerns however, since to cut welfare state expenditure would risk offending public opinion, that is, threaten its legitimation function: hence the presumed crisis, since, as Offe (1984, p.153) puts it, capitalism cannot survive without the welfare state, but cannot survive with it.

While neo-Marxist theory is of little help to us in explaining our material concerning health care priorities, resource allocation and managerial relations (which, we argued in the preceding section, are best explained by neo-élite theory), the fit with our material on funding (to which market relations are, of course, closely related) is quite good. We noted in Chapter 2 how demographic and technological changes had, amongst other things, led to increasing demand for NHS resources, demand which clashed with government economic priorities. We also saw in Chapter 3 the role of the CBI in lobbying for reductions in the NHS workforce.

The consistency of neo-Marxist theory with this material is even greater if one extends the theory a little. one obvious objection that can be made to the 'crisis of the welfare state' literature is that the imminence, or even the probability, of such a crisis would depend on the relationship between welfare state expenditure and the 'quantity' of legitimacy which it purchases. Such a relationship need not be linear; it might be possible to delay or avoid the crisis by purporting to increase the efficiency of the welfare state. In other words, if extended services can seem to be given without increases in expenditure, both capitalists and the public will be happy. We say 'seem' because, in this argument it is only perceptions that matter. (For an extended account of this argument, see Harrison, 1988a, pp.111-13.) It is a moot point as to whether the hypothesized crisis can be avoided indefinitely by such tactics; neo-Marxists would presumably argue that it cannot, but, as our concluding section shows, we are less certain.

Much of our material concerning NHS management structures (Chapter 3) can also be interpreted along the above lines; efficiency savings, cost-improvement programmes, performance indicators, general management, and internal markets are a succession of attempts to satisfy demands for additional resources by promising greater output without significantly greater input (Harrison, 1990). It is, of course, this last point which makes the link back from neo-Marxist theory to neo-élite theory, a linkage which we can now explore.

Explaining health policy

In the preceding two sections we have tried to show that the examples of health policy which we have examined can best be explained by a combination of two different theoretical approaches, neo-élite and neo-Marxist. These approaches are not, however, simply additive; rather, they relate to each other in a hierarchical fashion. Neo-Marxist theory has a higher level of generality ('comprehensiveness' is the term that we used in Chapter 1), and hence can be used to explain the consistency, or lack of it, of other less general theories at particular points in time. Thus, we reach the conclusion that neo-Marxist theory can be used to account for the shift from ideological corporatism to competition amongst structural interests in the period 1981 to 1984. In other words, economic factors have ultimately produced a modification in the structure of élites: a growing managerial challenge to the dominance of consultants, which is likely in its turn to bring about a weakening of the latter.

We do not, of course, claim that our analysis is complete and comprehensive. First, we have not undertaken an exhaustive examination of all aspects of health policy; in order to write a book of readable (and purchasable!) length we have omitted policies as important as health care and treatment practices, and relations with the pharmaceutical industry. Our conclusions hold only for the topics examined in Chapters 2 to 5, though we would defend this choice of topics not only on the grounds of their self-evident importance, but by pointing out that they are the ones which have tended to be the subject of the literature from which we derived the 'shared version' with which to contrast our own theoretical account.

Second, even within the scope of our material, neo-élite and neo-Marxist theories do not explain everything. Some important changes, such as the introduction of general management, sprang from the actions of individuals and to this extent are quite unanalysable in terms of any of the theoretical approaches which we have reviewed in this book. (The same is true of some highly visible – but within the terms of this book insubstantial – matters, such as differences in political party ideology, and intra-UK organizational differences.) This does not mean, however, that such changes might not be the appropriate subject of some other theory, which would be less general than neo-élite, but might relate to it in the same kind of hierarchical fashion as neo-élite theory does to neo-Marxist theory.

The notion that policy cannot be explained solely in terms of any one theory is not at all new (see, for instance, Klein, 1974b, pp.219–20), and indeed several authors have specifically endorsed the use of hierarchically ordered sets of theories to explain health and other social policies (see, for instance, Ham and Hill, 1984; Ham, 1985; Hambleton, 1986). There has, however, been little consensus about how to operationalize such a procedure, and our own approach has been more detailed and specific than that of others. We hope that it will serve as a foundation for further work of the same type both in health and other areas of social policy.

The future

Prior to about 1981, in most of the areas of health policy that we have examined, the government was not merely pulling punches, but not even fighting. When it did choose to enter the fray, on issues directly related to the total funding of the service, it was decisive. But in the early 1980s, other issues, such as resource allocation policy, management structures and clinical freedom, came to have potential effects on funding, so that the government is now fighting on these issues too.

This pervasive government involvement in the NHS has some implications for the future, which we shall conclude by addressing, though briefly and speculatively. It should be noted that, on our analysis, a change of government may not be very important, though it would certainly result in some changes (Cook, 1988); this is because any government is likely to have to face the same economic circumstances as the present one.

It seems likely to us that implementation of the kinds of measures proposed in *Working for Patients* will lead to further changes in the structure of the NHS élites. In particular, it seems possible that the differences of interest which will arise between purchasers and providers (see Annexe) in a situation of internal competition will form the focus for new élite cleavages, with perhaps some coalescence of medical and managerial élites within each. Further cleavage may occur if GPs and consultants find themselves in effective competition with each other. But all this assumes that the White Paper proposals will be implemented in letter and in spirit, that is, that there will be a substantial degree of genuine competition. As we write there are already signs that the government wishes to attenuate competition to some extent (Timmins, 1989, p.8).

We end our analysis by asking whether a government policy of staving off demands for additional health resources from one quarter and demands for reduced expenditure from another by purporting to improve the efficiency of the NHS can ultimately succeed. We believe that it is unlikely to do so. First, it seems unlikely to us that the *Working for Patients* proposals will result in significant net increases in efficiency, after such costs as additional management, information technology and possibly wasteful competition (Harrison, 1990) have been met. Second, and more crucially perhaps, the degree of adverse public opinion to which the White Paper proposals have given rise (see, for instance, Gaze, 1989, p.1233) suggest that any illusion of increasing efficiency may be difficult to sustain. Sooner or later, and whoever is in government, new policies for funding the NHS will have to be devised. If the basic analysis of neo-Marxist theory is correct, such policies will need to find some new way of changing the ratio between NHS spending and the 'quantity' of legitimacy which it purchases. One way of doing this would be to seek to undermine the NHS's own legitimacy in the public eye, with a view to its eventual dismantling; such a process of de-legitimatization is already discernable in other areas of the welfare state. The alternative would be an accommodation with capitalists at least to support the growth of the NHS in line with economic growth. We should like to see the latter, though this is not the same as saying that it is possible.

Annexe: The formal organization of the NHS

The following account of the formal organization of the National Health Service (NHS) is intended only to provide a working background against which the reader can understand the remainder of the book. In some cases, further detail can be found in Chapters 2 to 5, but on many details the reader will have to consult other literature. We have therefore provided a range of suitable references, though most will inevitably be out of date in respect of the changes arising from *Working for Patients*.

The following material is divided into a very brief account of the English NHS as it developed up to 1984, a slightly more detailed account of its organization at the time of the appearance of the White Paper *Working for Patients* in January 1989, and a summary of the changes proposed in that document. A further section summarizes the organizational variations found in the other countries of the United Kingdom, and we conclude the Annexe with speculations about future organizational developments. A list of abbreviations is appended. It should be remembered that the White Paper proposals are somewhat vague in many respects (*British Medical Journal*, vol.298, 1989, p.1167), and that even as we write (February 1990), clarifications emerge from the DoH and elsewhere; it is therefore difficult for us to be as confident in our analysis as we would wish.

1948–1984

The NHS came into existence in 1948, centrally funded (mainly from general taxation) and offering health care, free at the point of delivery, to the whole of the population. This source of funds remains unchanged today, as does entitlement to free services, except for the existence of charges (from which many are exempt) for items such as general practitioner (GP) prescriptions and general dental treatment. Until recently (see below) it has been an accepted principle that capital allocations did not have to be serviced, and that any unspent revenue had to be surrendered at the financial year end. (For accounts of the creation of the NHS, see Eckstein, 1960; Willcocks, 1967; Pater, 1981.) The Service remains the statutory responsibility of the relevant secretaries of state of the four component countries of the United Kingdom, whose departments (see below) are sometimes collectively referred to as the 'health departments'. In England, the Ministry of Health (founded in 1919) was subsumed in 1968 into the Department of Health and Social Security (DHSS), and separated out again in 1988 to become the Department of Health (DoH). Constitutionally, secretaries of state are responsible for the detailed provision of health services, not just (as, for instance, with nationalized industries) broad strategy. Consequently, quite detailed questions can be asked in Parliament, and select committees of the House of Commons (most notably the Committee of Public Accounts [PAC] and the Social Services Committee) have paid a good deal of attention to the NHS (Drewry, 1985; Garrett, 1986).

The original organizational structure of the NHS split responsibility between hospital authorities, local government authorities (responsible for community services), and executive councils (responsible for administering the contracts of – not managing – self-employed GPs, general dental practitioners, pharmacists and opticians). A degree of integration between the three parts of the Service was sought in 1974, when the NHS was reorganized; community services and hospital services became the responsibility of new health authorities (HAs), who also had some responsibility (via family practitioner committees – FPCs – successors to the executive councils) for the self-employed practitioners. HA boundaries were designed so as to approximate to local government boundaries, thus facilitating liaison with local authority social services departments. Other notable creations of the 1974 reorganizations were community health councils (CHCs) to represent the interests of health care consumers (for an account, see Klein and Lewis, 1976), four tiers of organization (department, region, area and district, in descending order), formalized multi-professional management through a system of management teams, whose decisions were to be reached by consensus (see Harrison, 1982; Schulz and Harrison, 1983), and a complex and comprehensive planning system (see Barnard et al, 1979). (A detailed account of developments in the formal organization of the NHS from 1948 to 1976 may be found in Harrison, 1988a, ch.2.)

Shortly afterwards, arrangements for the distribution (not the source) of funds were modified in two ways. After 1976, the system of volume financing, by which HAs were automatically compensated for increases in their costs (such as NHS pay or price rises) was replaced by the cash limits system which is now largely ubiquitous in the public services. (One major exception to this is the prescribing budget for GPs.) Secondly, the arrangements for allocating funds geographically between HAs were modified by the introduction of the resource allocation working party (RAWP) formula, with the intention of reducing historical inequities. The main elements of this formula (which is still ostensibly in use at the time of writing) are population size with adjustments for age, sex, standardized mortality ratios (the latter as a proxy for need), and for the flow of patients across HA boundaries. Implementation of this formula has always been difficult, since, at times of resource constraint (see Chapter 2), equity would have meant real cuts in funding for some HAs, and such equity has never, in fact been achieved, though variations have been reduced. Moreover, the formula has only been used consistently at regional level, with many sub-regional variations. (For more detailed accounts, see, for instance, Mays, 1987; Buxton and Klein, 1978.)

From 1981 onwards, managerial and organizational change in the NHS quickened in pace, with the introduction of performance indicators (PIs), the review process, compulsory competitive tendering for hospital support services, and the abolition of the area tier of organization (Harrison, 1988a, pp.56–63; for a complete account of the NHS as it existed around 1982, see Levitt and Wall, 1984). This process culminated in the changes which resulted from the first Griffiths Report (NHS Management Inquiry, 1983; for an account of the circumstances which led to this, see Harrison, 1988a, pp.60–1, 100–4 and Chapter 3 above).

1984–1989

Figure A 1 presents an outline of the organizational structure of the NHS in England as it existed immediately prior to the publication in early 1989 of the White Paper *Working for Patients*.

Within the DoH and chaired by the secretary of state were a health services supervisory board, whose function was to set overall objectives and broad strategy for the Service, and an NHS management board, whose role was to see to the implementation of these. (For a brief empirical account of the impact of these bodies, see Harrison, Hunter, Marnoch and Pollitt, 1989a, pp.7–8.) Both bodies were created on the recommendation of the Griffiths Report (NHS Management Inquiry, 1983), though the chairmanship arrangements represent a departure both from the original proposals and from subsequent modifications (Harrison, 1988a, pp.63–5; for details of board membership, see Chaplin, 1988, p.2). Below departmental level, England is divided into fourteen regions, each the responsibility of a regional health authority (RHA), and the regions are divided into a total of 190 districts, each the responsibility of a district health authority (DHA). The latter are responsible for the provision of hospital and community health services (such as home nursing and school health), and their disposition is loosely based on the notion of a catchment territory for a district general hospital (DGH) providing basic acute services. (In practice, there are major departures from this principle, as well as considerable cross-boundary flows of patients.)

RHAs and DHAs are statutory corporate bodies, whose members are appointed (not elected) to serve on a part-time and (except in the case of chairpersons) honorary basis. DHAs always include at least one consultant, one GP, one nurse, one (non-NHS) trade unionist and several local government authority appointees. There is therefore a sharp constitutional distinction between those members (for an analysis of whose role, see Ham, 1986), and the salaried officers whom the HA employs. The one result of the Griffiths Report which has been seen as more far-reaching then all its others was the substitution of individual chief executives (known as general managers) for the consensus management teams referred to in the preceding section. Regional general managers (RGMs), district general managers (DGMs) and unit general managers (UGMs), who may be from any professional or managerial background (see Harrison, 1988a, table 4.1), are employed on short-term rolling contracts, the renewal of which is ultimately dependent on annual appraisals of their performance. Health Authority PI figures and the review of HAs' progress towards national objectives and priorities may also provide evidence which is used in such individual performance review (IPR). General managers may also receive performance related pay (PRP). (For an empirical account of the work of DGMs and UGMs, see Harrison, Hunter, Marnoch and Pollitt, 1989a, pp.5–6.) Although there is no formal responsibility of DGMs to RGMs, or of RGMs to the NHS management board, the effect of these performance appraisal mechanisms has very much been to create one on a *de facto* basis (Harrison, 1988a, pp.118–19).

As Figure A.1 shows, other HA staff are responsible to general managers, though the status of consultants, who are in most cases employed by RHAs rather than the DHAs in which they work, is often regarded as somewhat ambiguous in this respect. The main

168   The dynamics of British health policy

```
                    ┌─────────────┐     DEPARTMENT OF HEALTH
                    │ Secretary of│    ┌──────────────┐
                    │  State for  │────│Health Services│
                    │   Health    │    │  Supervisory │
                    └─────────────┘    │    Board     │
                           │           └──────────────┘
                    ┌─────────────┐    ┌──────────────┐
                    │   Minister  │    │     NHS      │
                    │  for Health │────│  Management  │
                    └─────────────┘    │    Board     │
                                       └──────────────┘
┌──────────┐              │
│  Family  │              │
│Practitioner│            │
│Committees│              │
└──────────┘              │
      │                   │
┌──────────┐ ┌──────────┐ ┌──────────┐ ┌──────────┐
│ General  │ │Community │ │ Regional │ │ Regional │    ┌──────────┐
│ Medical  │ │  Health  │ │  Health  │─│ General  │────│ Regional │
│Pharmaceutical│ Councils │ │Authorities│ │ Manager │    │ Staff &  │
│ & Optical│ └──────────┘ └──────────┘ └──────────┘    │ Services │
│Practitioners│                  │                     └──────────┘
└──────────┘              ┌──────────┐ ┌──────────┐    ┌──────────┐
                          │ District │ │ District │    │ District │
                          │  Health  │─│ General  │────│    HQ    │
                          │Authorities│ │ Managers│    │   Staff  │
                          └──────────┘ └──────────┘    └──────────┘
                                       ┌──────────┐    ┌──────────┐
                                       │   Unit   │    │ Unit Staff│
                                       │ General  │────│ Hospital and│
                                       │ Managers │    │ Community│
                                       └──────────┘    │ Services │
                                                       └──────────┘
```

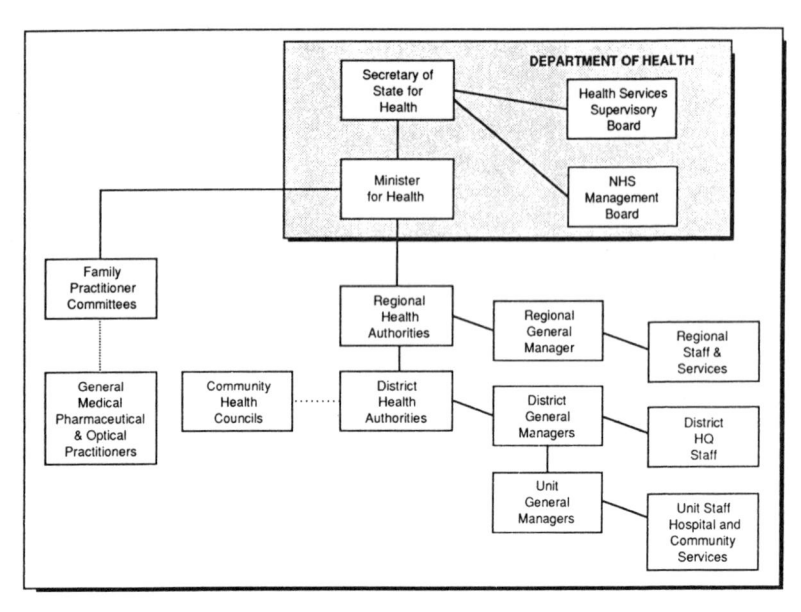

Figure A.1   Outline organizational structure of English NHS, *circa* 1988. *Source*: Adapted from S. Harrison, *Managing the National Health Service: Shifting the Frontier?* London, Chapman and Hall, 1988, fig. 4.1.

vehicle proposed by the Griffiths Report for handling the potentially rather difficult relationships between managers and doctors (see above, Chapter 4) was a system of 'management budgets' (MB, later re-styled as 'resource management', RM), in which clinical doctors were to receive workload-related budgets. Although such schemes have been (indeed, still are being) extensively piloted in the NHS, they have not yet been widely adopted. (For details, see Perrin, 1988; Pollitt *et al*, 1988; Buxton *et al*, 1989; Pinch *et al*, 1989.)

Finally, family practitioner committees (FPCs) continued to be somewhat less than fully integrated into the remainder of the NHS, having since 1985 been directly responsible to the DoH, and, despite the beginnings of more proactive managerial behaviour, continued to function mainly as servants of the self-employed practitioners. (For an empirical review, see Allsop and May, 1986.)

Working for patients: proposals for further reorganization

The intellectual basis of *Working for Patients* (Department of Health *et al*, 1989b), which appears to owe a good deal to the ideas of Enthoven (1985), is the assumption that a system of internal markets, in which NHS health care institutions compete with each other, will produce both greater efficiency and greater responsiveness to users. (For a detailed assessment of the White Paper, see Harrison, Hunter, Johnston and Wistow, 1989; Social Services Committee, 1989.) The creation of such an internal market entails the separation of two functions which are at present conflated in the role of DHAs: the provision of hospital and community health services, entailing the ownership of health care institutions and the employment of direct care staff, and the purchase (or commissioning) of care, that is, the allocation of funds to providing institutions so as to ensure that the needs of a population are met.

Before we describe the intended dynamics of the proposed internal market, we summarize the institutional changes designed to underpin it. It should be noted that the White Paper applies to the whole of the United Kingdom, although some institutional differences (such as the absence of regions outside England) and differences in nomenclature will remain. We have not referenced· each point of what follows; the most important sources are, of course, *Working for Patients* itself (Department of Health *et al*, 1989b) and associated Working Papers, together with a later document on self-governing hospitals (Department of Health, 1989b).

At the national level, within DoH, there will be a policy board and an NHS management executive with functions akin to, respectively, the former health services supervisory board and NHS management board (see above). The policy board includes a number of prominent industrialists in a part-time capacity, while the executive is rather smaller than its predecessor (*NHS Management Bulletin*, no.21, 1989). The other health departments will have somewhat different arrangements (see below).

English RHAs will remain in existence, with a core role of ensuring the implementation of central government policy; they will accordingly acquire hierarchical authority over FPCs. RHAs' other role, as providers of common services to DHAs, will correspondingly diminish. The membership of RHAs and DHAs (see below) will be modified in a way which ends the present sharp distinction between members and officers, since salaried chief officers of HAs will become 'executive' members of the authority itself, along with an equal number of part-time 'non-executives' and a chairperson. There will no longer be reserved places for the health care professions (see above), trades unionists, or local authority representatives, and the new authorities will resemble the boards of directors of commercial organizations.

The primary role of DHAs and their equivalents outside England will be to *purchase* health care for their *resident* population, implying that cross-boundary patient flows will entail financial transfers between DHAs, rather than the elaborate retrospective adjustments to allocation targets which are entailed in the present RAWP arrangements. It is also expected that DHAs will not be involved in the day-to-day management of the institutions that they own, but rather relate to them through quasi-contractual 'management budgets'. (We discuss this in more detail below.)

Turning to health care institutions themselves (the White Paper uses the term 'hospital' to embrace all kinds of these, including community health services), a system of charging for capital funds (including for the value of existing assets) will be introduced in order to allow fair competition between institutions. The present series of RM pilot schemes will be extended to additional institutions. Consultant contracts of employment will specify their duties in greater detail, accompanied by detailed local job descriptions, and their participation in medical audit will be compulsory. The role of hospitals in the education and training of health care professionals will be funded separately from the mechanism of allocating funds for patient care.

Perhaps the most controversial of the *Working for Patients* proposals is that institutions will be able to apply to the secretary of state to become 'self-governing', that is to be released from ownership by a DHA. Such NHS Hospital Trusts, once established (with membership analogous to that of DHAs) will have a number of freedoms not available to other institutions. The most important of these will be freedom from Whitley Council and other nationally determined terms and conditions of service (see Chapter 4, above), and the freedom to accumulate financial year-end surpluses for re-investment, though it appears that capital charges will be set so as to return a proportion of such surpluses to the government.

The White Paper's proposals for primary care services owe something to an earlier White Paper *Promoting Better Health* (DHSS *et al*, 1987). As noted above, FPCs will be integrated into the remainder of NHS management by becoming accountable to RHAs. Proposed changes in FPC membership will give the self-employed practitioners a less prominent role, and the FPC will acquire a more explicit managerial role than at present, including rights to receive information about prescribing and hospital referral patterns and will be re-designated Family Health Service Authority. Individual general practices will receive 'indicative' prescribing budgets rather than cash limits, but will have to justify any expenditure over budget. Controversial changes to the relative importance of different elements of GP income are to be made; capitation fees (received in respect of each patient on a GP's list) will increase in importance while basic practice allowances will decrease, and fees for individual vaccinations and cervical smears will be replaced by payments for reaching a specified target coverage of relevant patients. The intention in all this is to provide a greater incentive for GPs to attract patients and to widen the coverage of preventive measures. GPs, like hospital consultants, will be required to participate in medical audit.

Another controversial White Paper proposal is that larger general practices can opt to receive 'practice funds' from the RHA. Such a budget would include the elements for prescribing and grants for staff salaries and premises improvements received by ordinary practices, in addition to an amount reflecting the practice's potential hospital referrals to outpatients, to pathology and X-ray, and for specified elective surgical procedures. (The amount of the last element would correspondingly be deducted from the RHA's allocation to the relevant DHAs.) Practice fund-holders would not, however, be required to employ the various elements of the budget in accordance with the original basis of calculation (for instance, a GP would be able to undertake minor surgery in order to save a hospital referral), and unspent allocations would remain within the practice.

Figure A.2 is not a conventional organization chart but rather an attempt to illustrate the intended dynamics of the new system. It should be noted that for simplicity we have omitted a number of considerations (such as special health authorities, and supra-regional specialties), and ignored the immense complications of the proposed transitional period. The figure therefore illustrates the intended 1992-3 endpoint of the reorganization process.

It is evident from Figure A.2 that the proposed market might consist of up to four different types of institution competing for the resources of a particular DHA or practice fund-holding GP. Arrangements between a DHA and private sector hospitals, self-governing NHS trusts or units owned by a different DHA will be contractual, as will arrangements between fund-holding GPs and all institutions. (Except in the case of the private sector, there will be arbitration arrangements to deal with disputes.) In the case of a DHA's directly managed unit, the relationship will be a management budget, a quasi-contract with similar provisions to commercial contracts (see below), since the intention is that DHAs should not be so closely involved in the management of hospitals as is presently the case. The figure clearly illustrates the separation of purchasing and provision which, as we noted above, is the basis of the market.

The proposed system rests heavily on the assumption that DHAs and fund-holding GPs will be prepared to commit resources prospectively to meet the anticipated health needs of their population or patients, retaining only a relatively small proportion of funds for contingencies. For some 'core' services, such as accident and emergency, or immediate medical and surgical admissions, contracts will necessarily be let locally, though not necessarily within the DHA's boundaries. (The precise definition of 'core' is for local determination.) Other services ('where patients and their GPs have time to choose when and where to seek hospital treatment': Department of Health *et al*, 1989b, para.4.19) may be the subject of contracts with hospitals in any location. Contracts (and management budgets) will need to specify the type of patient or procedure involved, the standards to which treatment will be given (implying a quality control mechanism: see Chapter 5), and a basis of price. Most contracts will also be expected to specify the numbers of cases or level of service over which they will apply.

Caring for people: proposals for community care reform

In November 1989, the government published its long-awaited plans in response to the proposals for reforming community care which we outlined in Chapter 3. The latest White Paper, *Caring for People* (Department of Health *et al*, 1989b), is concerned with the care in their own homes (or in 'homely' settings in the community) of people who are elderly, mentally ill or mentally handicapped, and those with physical or sensory disabilities. The document endeavours to distinguish between 'social care', including such services as home helps, aids and adaptations for the disabled, residential and nursing home care, day care, respite care and adult training centres, and 'health care'. The latter will continue to be the responsibility of health authorities, including the provision of long stay residential health care for the highly dependent, the assessment of mentally ill people prior to discharge into social care, the coordination of hospice care, and the

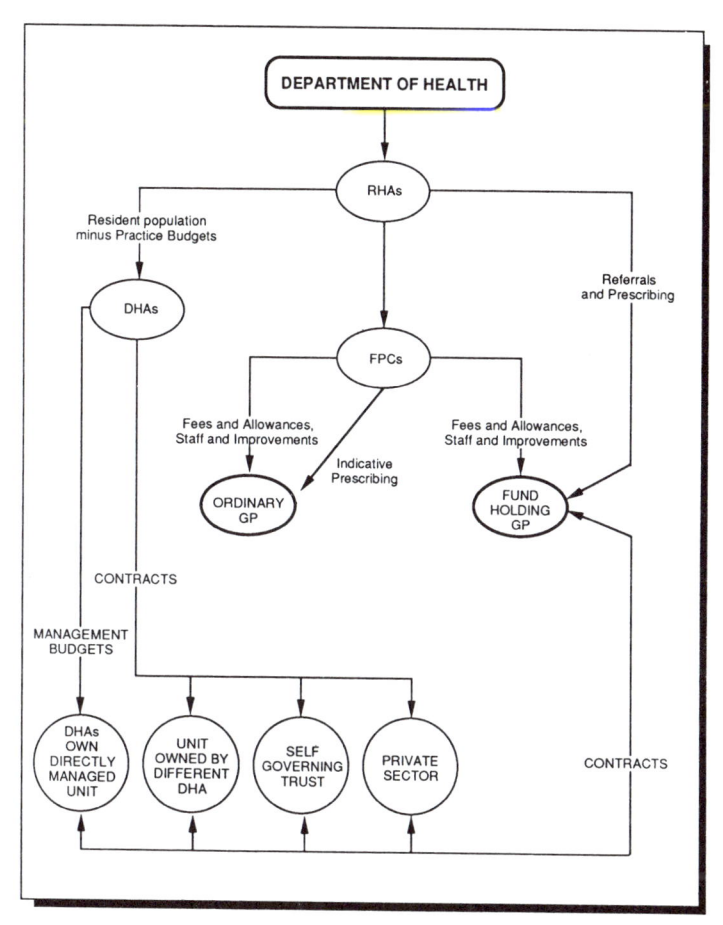

Figure A.2 Proposed major NHS funding flows, 1992–3.

provision of health-related professional advice to local government authorities.

Local authorities will be responsible for social care, employing, in addition to existing funds, resources made available from the NHS (these have yet to be determined; the only 'ring-fenced' element will be a specific mental illness grant channelled via RHAs) and from the social security system (a unified social care budget channelled via the revenue support grant). Local authorities will be required to engage in community care planning and to establish and publish their referral and entry procedures, and criteria for access, to social care. Particularly dependent clients will be expected to have a 'case manager' (usually, though not necessarily, employed by the local authority Social Services Department) responsible for orchestrating the various inputs to the individual. It is possible that case managers will be budget holders, but in any event, the White Paper aims to shift the emphasis of local authority activity away from direct provision, and towards a 'purchaser' role somewhat analogous to that envisaged for DHAs in the earlier White Paper. Consequently, case managers will be able to choose between local authority and private residential care and domiciliary care. This model is buttressed by changes in the social security regulations aimed, firstly, at removing the perverse incentives towards residential care (which we outlined in Chapter 3), secondly, at making the use of private sector residential accommodation financially more attractive to local authorities, and thirdly, at encouraging the provision of home-based care where appropriate.

Wales, Scotland and Northern Ireland

Because textbook descriptions often concentrate upon the English NHS, it is often mistakenly assumed that a uniform structure applies throughout the United Kingdom. In fact, the NHS in Wales, Scotland and Northern Ireland has been administratively devolved to the Welsh Office, Scottish Office and Northern Ireland Office respectively. The NHS in each of these three countries is the political responsibility of the relevant secretary of state, usually assisted by a junior minister. Consequently, some differences in policymaking, as well as structure, are evident. (For a more detailed discussion in respect of Wales and Scotland, see Hunter, 1984 and Hunter and Wistow, 1987; 1988; for Northern Ireland, see Hunter, 1982; Birrell and Williamson, 1983; Connolly, 1985.)

The most notable difference in Wales, Scotland and Northern Ireland is the absence of a regional tier of organization. This was removed at the time of the 1974 reorganization and replaced with a common services agency function, located at the centre in each country, but jointly-managed by government and health service. The three other United Kingdom health departments perform some of the functions which in England would be part of the regional role, while health authorities perform others. This has resulted in a different style of policymaking and quality of centre–periphery relationship from those found in England. Moreover, the scale of operation is quite different; there are nine DHAs in Wales, fifteen health boards in Scotland, and four health and social services boards in Northern Ireland.

Two other major structural differences are worth noting. First, in Northern Ireland the health and social services are structurally integrated, which is unique in the United Kingdom (Connolly, 1985). Second, in Scotland and Northern Ireland there are no separate FPCs administering GP (and other) services; these come under the control of the Boards, thus offering a degree of integration not evident in England and Wales.

Other, more subtle, differences are evident in the resource allocation formulae, variants of RAWP, devised for the three countries, and in the approaches adopted to health planning. For instance, the Scottish Health Service Planning Council which existed from 1974 to 1989 had no equivalent elsewhere (Wiseman, 1979). Similarly, the Welsh Health Planning Forum established in 1988 has no counterpart. Both the Planning Council in Scotland (and its successor the Advisory Council) and the Planning Forum in Wales, while displaying some differences, exist to provide independent advice to the secretary of state.

Since the Griffiths Report of 1983 (NHS Management Inquiry, 1983), changes in management arrangements for Wales, Scotland and Northern Ireland have, broadly, followed those in England. The major difference has been in timing, England having been made to take a lead role. But other important differences are evident. Most notably, at the time of the introduction of general management in 1984, Northern Ireland did not appoint general managers at unit level, instead retaining unit management groups. In Northern Ireland also, there have been no changes in the central health department equivalent to those elsewhere, and a chief executive for the Northern Ireland NHS has only recently been appointed. The present incumbent is a career civil servant, which also sets Northern Ireland apart from England, Wales and Scotland, though the latter has only recently come into line with England and Wales, where chief executives have prior experience of health service management.

In Wales, the NHS functions under the strategic direction of the Health Policy Board, chaired by the secretary of state; this is equivalent to the policy board (formerly the supervisory board) in England. An executive committee of the board is led by the director (i.e. chief executive) of the NHS in Wales, and is responsible for implementing the board's decisions. These arrangements, introduced in 1984, will remain unaffected by *Working for Patients*.

In Scotland, a health service policy board established in 1985 has been abolished as a result of the White Paper. The reason given is that 'Broad issues of policy can be dealt with more effectively by ministers directly, seeking advice as necessary through meetings with representatives of health boards and other bodies and, in future, through the work of the Advisory Council' (Department of Health et al, 1989b, para.10.18). Scotland has not until recently adopted the kind of review process evident in England, having instead a round of (rather ineffective) bi-annual reviews. However, it has now been decided that the new chief executive will initiate an annual round of target-setting and accountability reviews of health boards, though it is not yet clear whether ministers will be involved. Moves are also now underway to introduce resource management to Scotland, which is seen in this respect to have lagged behind England. Changes at the centre in Northern Ireland have not so far been proposed though, as we noted above, a chief executive has been appointed.

The future of NHS organization: a concluding comment

We close our description of NHS organization by drawing attention to two probable medium-term developments, both of which seem likely to result from the *Working for Patients* proposals. First, the greater the number of institutions that become self-governing, the smaller the residual role in managing services that will remain for DHAs, and the more they will be able to concentrate on their purchasing function. Mergers of neighbouring DHAs would then be a logical next step (Department of Health et al, 1989b, para.3.20), providing greater market power for purchasers in relation to providers. Second, it would also become attractive to merge FPCs and DHAs, giving the latter a degree of influence over the (non-budget holding) GPs for whose hospital referrals they are financially responsible. Any possible developments, and indeed the implementation of existing proposals, must of course be contemplated in the knowledge that a general election must occur before 1992, though the implications of this are not at all clear.

List of abbreviations

BMA	British Medical Association
BUPA	British United Provident Association
CEPOD	Confidential Enquiry into Perioperative Deaths
CHC	Community Health Council
CIP	Cost-improvement Programme
CMC	Central Manpower Committee
DHSS	Department of Health and Social Security
DoH	Department of Health
DHA	District Health Authority
FPC	Family Practitioner Committee
FPS	Family Practitioner Services
GDP	Gross Domestic Product
GMC	General Medical Council
GP	General [Medical] Practitioner
HA	Health Authority
HAS	Health Advisory Service
HCHS	Hospital and Community Health Services
HFA 2000	Health For All by the Year 2000
IHSM	Institute of Health Services Management
IPR	Individual Performance Review
JCC	Joint Consultants Committee
JPAC	Joint [Manpower] Planning Advisory Committee
NAHA	National Association of Health Authorities in England and Wales
NALGO	National and Local Government Officers' Association
NHS	National Health Service
OPCS	Office of Population Censuses and Surveys
PESC	Public Expenditure Survey Committee
PI	Performance Indicator
PMA	Partisan Mutual Adjustment (Lindblom)
PRP	Performance Related Pay
PSBR	Public Sector Borrowing Requirement
RHA	Regional Health Authority
RAWP	Resource Allocation Working Party
RM	Resonne Management
RCGP	Royal College of General Practitioners
RCN	Royal College of Nursing
SHAPE	*Scottish Health Authorities Priorities for the Eighties* (SHHD, 1980)
SHARPEN	*Scottish Health Authorities Review of Priorities for the Eighties and Nineties* (SHHD, 1988)
SHO	Senior House Officer
SR	Senior Registrar
WHO	World Health Organization

References

ADVISORY COMMITTEE FOR MEDICAL MANPOWER PLANNING (1985), Report (London: DHSS).
ALFORD, R. R. (1975), *Health Care Politics* (Chicago: University of Chicago Press).
ALLSOP, J. (1984), *Health Policy and the National Health Service* (London: Longman).
ALLSOP, J. and MAY, A. (1986), *The Emperor's New Clothes: Family Practitioner Committees in the 1980s* (London: King Edward's Hospital Fund for London).
ANDERSON, D., LAIT, J. and MARSLAND, D. (1981), *Breaking the Spell of the Welfare State* (London: Social Affairs Unit).
APPLEYARD, W. J. (1976), 'Hospital medical staffing', *British Medical Journal*, vol. 1, pp.136–7.
APPLEYARD, W. J. (1982), 'Medical manpower mismanagement: mirage or miracle?', *British Medical Journal*, vol. 284, pp.1351–5.
ASCHER, K. (1987), *The Politics of Privatisation: Contracting Out Public Services* (London: Macmillan).
AUDIT COMMISSION (1986), *Making a Reality of Community Care* (London: Audit Commission).
BACHRACH, P. and BARATZ, M. S. (1970), *Power and Poverty: Theory and Practice* (London: Oxford University Press).
BAIN, G. S. and ELSHEIK, F. (1976), *Trade Union Growth and The Business Cycle* (Oxford: Blackwell).
BARNARD, K. and HARRISON, S. (1986), 'Labour relations in health services management', *Social Science and Medicine*, vol. 22, no.11, pp.1213–28.
BARNARD, K., LEE, K., MILLS, A. and REYNOLDS, J. (1979), *Towards a New Rationality: a Study of Planning in the NHS* (in four volumes) (University of Leeds: Nuffield Centre for Health Services Studies).
BERNSTEIN, R. J. (1976), *The Restructuring of Social and Political Theory* (London: Methuen).
BIRCH, S. and MAYNARD, A. (1986), 'Equalising access to health within the UK', *Public Money*, vol. 6, no.2, pp.54–5.
BIRRELL, D. and WILLIAMSON, A. (1983), 'Northern Ireland's integrated health and personal social service structure' in A. Williamson and G. Room (eds), *Health and Welfare States of Britain: An Inter-Country Comparison* (London: Heinemann).
BOSANQUET, N. (ed.) (1979), *Industrial Relations in the NHS: the Search for a System* (London: King's Fund).

BOSANQUET, N. (1985), *Public Expenditure Rules and the NHS*, Discussion Paper No.3 (York: University of York Centre for Health Economics).
BRAND, C. and McGILL, I. (1978), *A Review of East Sussex AHA Machinery for Joint Consultation* (Brighton: Brighton Polytechnic).
BROWN, R. G. S. (1975), *The Management of Welfare* (London: Fontana).
BROWN, R. G. S. (1979), *Reorganising the National Health Service: A Case Study of Administrative Charge* (Oxford: Blackwell and Martin Robertson).
BROWN, R. G. S., GRIFFIN, S. and HAYWOOD, S. C. (1975), *New Bottles: Old Wine?* (Hull: University of Hull Institute for Health Studies).
BUCK, N., DEVLIN, B. and LUNN, J. N. (1987), *Report of a Confidential Enquiry Into Perioperative Deaths* (London: Nuffield Provincial Hospitals Trust).
BURNS, T. (1981), *Rediscovering Organisation: Aspects of Collaboration and Managerialism in Hospital Organisation*, unpublished review.
BUTLER, J. R. and VAILE, M. S. B. (1984), *Health and Health Services: An Introduction to Health Care in Britain* (London: Routledge and Kegan Paul).
BUXTON, M. J. and KLEIN, R. E. (1978), *Allocating Health Resources: A Commentary on the Report of the Resource Allocation Working Party*, Royal Commission on the National Health Service, Research Paper no.3 (London: HMSO).
BUXTON, M., PACKWOOD, T. and KEEN, J. (1989), *Resource Management: Process and Progress* (London: Department of Health).
CARPENTER, M. (1985), *They Still Go Marching On – A Celebration of COHSE's First Seventy-five Years* (London: Confederation of Health Service Employees).
CASTLE, B. (1980), *The Castle Diaries 1974–76* (London: Weidenfeld and Nicolson).
CAWSON, A. (1982), *Corporatism and Welfare: Social Policy and State Intervention in Britain* (London: Heinemann Educational Books).
CAWSON, A. (1985), 'Varieties of Corporatism: the importance of the meso-level of interest intermediation' in A. Cawson (ed.), *Organised Interests and the State: Studies in Meso-Corporatism* (London: Sage).
CBI WORKING PARTY ON GOVERNMENT EXPENDITURE (1981), *Report* (London: Confederation of British Industry).
CENTRAL STATISTICAL OFFICE (1986), *Regional Trends 21* (London: HMSO).
CHAPLIN, N. W. (ed.) (1988), *The Hospitals and Health Services Yearbook and Directory of Hospital Suppliers* (London: Institute of Health Services Management).
CLEGG, H. A. and CHESTER, T. E. (1957), *Wage Policy and the National Health Service* (Oxford: Blackwell).
COCHRANE, A. L. (1972), *Effectiveness and Efficiency: Random Reflections on Health Services* (London: Nuffield Provincial Hospitals Trust).
COMMITTEE OF ENQUIRY INTO THE COST OF THE NATIONAL HEALTH SERVICE (1956), (Chairman: Mr. C. W.

Guillebaud), *Report*, Cmnd.663 (London: HMSO).
COMMITTEE OF PUBLIC ACCOUNTS (1981), *Seventeenth Report, Session 1980–81: Financial Control and Accountability in the National Health Service* (London: House of Commons/HMSO).
COMMITTEE OF PUBLIC ACCOUNTS (1982), *Seventeenth Report, Session 1981–82: Financial Control and Accountability in the National Health Service; Cost of Remedying Defects in Hospitals; Working Practices in the National Health Service* (London: House of Commons/HMSO).
CONNOLLY, M. (1985), 'Integrating health and social services: has the Northern Ireland experiment succeeded?', *Public Money*, vol. 4, no.4, pp.263–300.
COOK, R. (1988), *Questions of Health: A Labour Green Paper on Health Policy* (London: Labour Party).
CIPFA (1987), *Health Service Trends vol. 1: The CIPFA Database* (London: Chartered Institute of Public Finance and Accountancy).
CROSSMAN, R. H. S. (1977), *The Diaries of a Cabinet Minister: Volume 3; Secretary of State for Social Services 1968–1970* (London: Hamish Hamilton and Jonathan Cape).
CROUCH, C. (1983), 'Pluralism and the new corporatism', *Political Studies*, vol. xxxi, no.1, pp.86–102.
DAHL, R. A. (1985), *A Preface to Economic Democracy* (Cambridge: Polity Press).
DAVIES, C. (1987), 'Viewpoint: things to come: the NHS in the next decade', *Sociology of Health and Illness*, vol. 9, no.3, pp.302–17.
DAVIES, P. (1986), 'BMA – iron fist in a velvet glove', *Health Service Journal*, 11 December, p.1603.
DAVIES, P. (1989), 'The NHS goes to the opinion polls', *Health Service Journal*, 22 June, pp.750–1.
DAY, P. and KLEIN, R. E. (1987), *Accountabilities: Five Public Services* (London: Tavistock).
DAY, P., KLEIN, R. E. and TIPPING, G. (1988), *Inspecting for Quality: Services for the Elderly*, Social Policy Paper no.12 (Bath: University of Bath Centre for Social Policy).
DEPARTMENT OF EMPLOYMENT (1987), *New Earnings Survey* (London: HMSO).
DEPARTMENT OF HEALTH (1989a), *Kenneth Clarke's Statement to Parliament on the Future Arrangements for Community Care*, 12 July.
DEPARTMENT OF HEALTH (1989b), *Self-Governing Hospitals: An Initial Guide* (London: HMSO).
DEPARTMENT OF HEALTH AND SOCIAL SECURITY (1976), *Priorities for the Health and Personal Social Services in England* (London: HMSO).
DEPARTMENT OF HEALTH AND SOCIAL SECURITY (1977), *Annual Report of the Health Advisory Service for the Year 1976* (London: HMSO).
DEPARTMENT OF HEALTH AND SOCIAL SECURITY (1979), 'If industrial relations break down', Circular HC(79)20 (London).
DEPARTMENT OF HEALTH AND SOCIAL SECURITY (1981), *Report of a Study on Community Care* (London).

DEPARTMENT OF HEALTH AND SOCIAL SECURITY (1981), 'Plans to double the numbers of consultants in fifteen years', Press Release no.81/184 (London).
DEPARTMENT OF HEALTH AND SOCIAL SECURITY (1982a), *Government Response to the Fourth Report from the Social Services Committee 1980–81*, Cmnd.8479 (London: HMSO).
DEPARTMENT OF HEALTH AND SOCIAL SECURITY (1982b), 'Health services management – hospital medical staff career structure and training', Circular HC(82)4 (London).
DEPARTMENT OF HEALTH AND SOCIAL SECURITY (1983), *Health Care and Its Costs: the Development of the National Health Service in England* (London: HMSO).
DEPARTMENT OF HEALTH AND SOCIAL SECURITY (1985), 'Joint Planning of Medical and Dental Training Grades in the NHS and Universities', Press Release no. 85/333 (London).
DEPARTMENT OF HEALTH AND SOCIAL SECURITY (1986), *Government Response to the Fifth Report from the Social Services Committee 1984–85 Session* (London: HMSO).
DEPARTMENT OF HEALTH AND SOCIAL SECURITY (1987), *Health and Personal Social Services Statistics for England: 1987 Edition* (London: HMSO).
DEPARTMENT OF HEALTH AND SOCIAL SECURITY (NORTHERN IRELAND) (1975), *Strategy for the Development of Health and Personal Social Services in Northern Ireland* (Belfast: HMSO).
DEPARTMENT OF HEALTH AND SOCIAL SECURITY AND WELSH OFFICE (1979), *Patients First: Consultative Paper on the Structure and Management of the National Health Service in England and Wales* (London: HMSO).
DEPARTMENT OF HEALTH AND SOCIAL SECURITY, WELSH OFFICE, NORTHERN IRELAND OFFICE AND SCOTTISH OFFICE (1987), *Promoting Better Health: the Government's Programme for Improving Primary Health Care* (London: HMSO).
DEPARTMENT OF HEALTH, DEPARTMENT OF SOCIAL SECURITY, WELSH OFFICE AND SCOTTISH OFFICE (1989a) *Caring for People*, CM 849 (London: HMSO).
DEPARTMENT OF HEALTH, WELSH OFFICE, SCOTTISH HOME AND HEALTH DEPARTMENT, AND NORTHERN IRELAND OFFICE (1989b), *Working for Patients*, CM 555 (London: HMSO).
DEVLIN, H. B. (1988), 'Professional audit: quality control – keeping up to date', *Ballière's Clinical Anaesthiology*, vol. 2, no.2.
DIMMOCK, S. J. (1982), 'Incomes Policy and Health Services in the United Kingdom' in A. S. Sethi and S. J. Dimmock (eds), *Industrial Relations and Health Services* (London: Croom Helm).
DORAN, F. S. A. (1973), 'Expansion of the consultant grade', *British Medical Journal*, vol. 1, suppl., pp.71–4.
DOYLE, C. (1981), 'Junior doctors face the dole queue', *Observer*, 8 March.
DRAPER, P. and SMART, T. (1974), 'Social service and health policy in

the UK: some contributions of the social sciences to the bureaucratisation of the NHS', *International Journal of Health Services*, vol. 4, no.3, pp.453–70.
DREWRY, G. (ed.) (1985), *The New Select Committees: A Study of the 1979 Reforms* (Oxford: Clarendon Press).
DUNLEAVY, P. (1981), 'Professions and policy change: notes towards a model of ideological corporatism', *Public Administration Bulletin*, no.36, pp.3–16.
DUNLEAVY, P. (1989), 'The architecture of the British central state: Part 1: framework for analysis', *Public Administration*, vol. 67, no.3, pp.249–76.
DUNLEAVY, P. and O'LEARY, B. (1987), *Theories of the State: The Politics of Liberal Democracy* (London: Macmillan).
DUNSIRE, A., HARTLEY, K., PARKER, D., and DIMITRIOU, B. (1988), 'Organisational status and performance: testing public choice theories', *Public Administration*, vol. 66, no.4, pp.363–88.
DYSON, R. F. (1983), 'Pay noose for National Health Service?', *British Medical Journal*, vol. 286, pp.995–6.
DYSON, R. F. and SPARY, K. A. (1979), 'Professional associations' in N. Bosanquet (ed.), *Industrial Relations in the NHS: The Search for a System* (London: King's Fund Institute).
ECKSTEIN, H. (1960), *Pressure Group Politics: the Case of the British Medical Association* (London: Allen and Unwin).
ELCOCK, H. (1978), 'Regional government in action: the members of two regional health authorities', *Public Administration*, vol. 56, no.4, pp.379–98.
ELCOCK, H. and HAYWOOD, S. (1980), *The Buck Stops Where? Accountability and Control in the National Health Service* (Hull: University of Hull Institute for Health Studies).
ENGLEMAN, S. R. (1977), 'The hospital medical career structure', *Health Services Manpower Review*, vol. 3, no.4, pp.18–20.
ENGLEMAN, S. R. (1978), 'Hospital medical manpower planning', *Health and Social Service Journal*, Centre Eight Paper, pp.A1–A6.
ENTHOVEN, A. C. (1985), *Reflections on the Management of the National Health Service: an American looks at incentives to efficiency in health services management in the U.K.* (London: Nuffield Provincial Hospitals Trust).
EXPENDITURE COMMITTEE (1978), Selected Public Expenditure Programmes Chapter 5: Session 1977–78: Eighth Report, HC 600 (London: HMSO).
FEINMANN, J. (1988), 'London GP deputising is thrown into disarray', *Health Service Journal*, 4 February, p.144.
FORTE, P. G. L. (1986), *Decision-Making and Planning in a District Health Authority: A Review and a Case Study*, Working Paper no.466 (Leeds: University of Leeds School of Geography).
FOX, A. (1966), *Industrial Sociology and Industrial Relations*, Royal Commission on Trade Union and Employers' Associations, Research Paper no.3 (London: HMSO).
FOX, P. D. (1978), 'Managing Health Resources "English Style"' in G. McLachlan (ed.), *By Guess or By What? Information Without Design in the*

NHS (Oxford: Oxford University Press/Nuffield Provincial Hospitals Trust).
FRYER, R. H., FAIRCLOUGH, A. J. and MANSON, T. (1974), *Organisation and Change in NUPE* (London: National Union of Public Employees).
GARRETT, J. (1986), 'Developing State Audit in Britain', *Public Administration*, vol. 64, no.4, pp.421–33.
GAZE, H. (1989), 'Consumer groups step up patients' rights campaign', *Health Service Journal*, 12 October, p.1233.
GLENNERSTER, H., KORMAN, N., and MARSLEN-WILSON, F. (1983), 'Plans and practice: the participants' views', *Public Administration*, vol. 61, no.3, pp.253–64.
GODT, P. (1987), 'Confederation, consent, and corporatism: state strategies and the medical profession in France, Great Britain and West Germany', *Journal of Health Politics, Policy and Law*, vol. 12, no.3, pp.459–80.
GOLDSMITH, M. (1988), 'Do vouchers hold the key to the funding dilemma?' *Health Service Journal*, 21 January.
GOODIN, R. E. (1982), 'Rational politicians and rational bureaucrats in Washington and Whitehall', *Public Administration*, vol. 60, no.1, pp.23–41.
GRAY, A. and HUNTER, D. J. (1983), 'Priorities and resource allocation in the Scottish Health Service: some problems in planning and implementation', *Policy and Politics*, vol. 11, no.4, pp.417–37.
GRIFFITH, B. and RAYNER, G. (1985), *Commercial Medicine in London* (London: Greater London Council).
GRIFFITHS, R. (1987), 'Measuring Performance in the NHS' in *Performance Measurement and the Consumer* (London: National Consumer Council).
GRIFFITHS, R. (1988), *Community Care: Agenda for Action* (London: HMSO).
HALLAS, J. (1976), *CHCs in Action* (London: Nuffield Provincial Hospitals Trust).
HAM, C. J. (1980), 'Community Health Council Participation in the NHS Planning System', *Social Policy and Administration*, vol. 14, no.3, pp.221–231.
HAM, C. J. (1981), *Policy Making in the National Health Service* (London: Macmillan).
HAM, C. J. (1985), *Health Policy in Britain*, 2nd edition (London: Macmillan).
HAM, C. J. (1986), *Managing Health Services: Health Authority Members in Search of a Role* (Bristol: University of Bristol School for Advanced Urban Studies).
HAM, C. J. and HILL, M. J. (1984), *The Policy Process in the Modern Capitalist State* (Brighton, Sussex: Wheatsheaf).
HAM, C. J. and HUNTER, D. J. (1988), *Managing Clinical Activity in the NHS*, Briefing Paper no.8 (London: King's Fund Institute).
HAMBLETON, R. (1986), *Rethinking Policy Planning* (Bristol: University of Bristol School for Advanced Urban Studies).
HARRISON, S. (1981), 'The politics of health manpower' in A. F. Long

and G. Mercer (eds), *Manpower Planning in the National Health Service*, Farnborough: Gower Press).

HARRISON, S. (1982), 'Consensus decisionmaking in the National Health Service: a review', *Journal of Management Studies*, vol. 19, no.4, pp.377–94.

HARRISON, S. (1988a), *Managing the National Health Service: Shifting the Frontier?* (London: Chapman and Hall).

HARRISON, S. (1988b) 'The closed shop and the National Health Service: a case study in public sector labour relations', *Journal of Social Policy*, vol. 17, Pt.1, pp.61–81.

HARRISON, S. (1988c), 'The workforce and the new managerialism' in R. J. Maxwell (ed.), *Reshaping the National Health Service* (Hermitage, Berks: Policy Journals), pp.141–52.

HARRISON, S. (1989), 'Industrial relations at national level' in B. Connah and S. Lancaster (eds), *The National Health Service Handbook* (4th edition) (London: Macmillan/National Association of Health Authorities in England and Wales), pp.194–6.

HARRISON, S. (1990), 'Internal markets' in L. H. W. Paine (ed.), *Association of National Health Service Supplies Officers Members' Reference Book and Buyers Guide* (London: Sterling Publications).

HARRISON, A. and GRETTON, J. (1986) 'Are the government really spending more on the NHS?' in A. Harrison and J. Gretton (eds), *Health Care UK: 1986* (Hermitage, Berks: Policy Journals).

HARRISON, S. and LONG, A. F. (1989), 'Concepts of performance in medical care organisations', *Journal of Management in Medicine*, vol. 3, pp.176–92.

HARRISON, S. and SCHULZ, R. I. (1988), 'Impact of the Griffiths reforms of National Health Service management: the views of psychiatrists', *Health Services Management Research*, vol. 1, no.3, pp.127–34.

HARRISON, S., HAYWOOD, S., and FUSSELL, C. (1984), 'Problems and solutions: the perceptions of NHS managers', *Hospital and Health Services Review*, vol. 80, no.4.

HARRISON, S., HUNTER, D. J., JOHNSTON, I. and WISTOW, G. (1989), *Competing for Health: A Commentary on the NHS Review* (Leeds: University of Leeds Nuffield Institute for Health Services Studies).

HARRISON, S., HUNTER, D. J., MARNOCH, G. and POLLITT, C. J. (1989a), *The Impact of General Management in the NHS: Before and After the White Paper*, Nuffield Institute Report no. 2 (Leeds: University of Leeds Nuffield Institute for Health Services Studies).

HARRISON, S., HUNTER, D. J., MARNOCH, G. and POLLITT, C. J. (1989b), 'General management and medical autonomy in the National Health Service', *Health Services Management Research*, vol. 2, no.1.

HAYEK, F. A. von (1986), *The Road to Serfdom* (London: Routledge).

HAYWOOD, S. C. (1979), 'Team management in the NHS: what is it all about?', *Health and Social Service Journal*, Centre 8 Paper, 5 October.

HAYWOOD, S. C. and ALASZEWSKI, A. (1980), *Crisis in the Health Service: the Politics of Management* (London: Croom Helm).

HAYWOOD, S. C. and HUNTER, D. J. (1982), 'Consultative

processes in health policy in the United Kingdom: a view from the centre', *Public Administration*, vol. 60, no.2, pp.143–62.

HECLO, H. and WILDAVSKY, A. (1981), *The Private Government of Public Money* (2nd edition) (London: Macmillan).

HELD, D. (1987), *Models of Democracy* (Cambridge: Polity Press).

HELLER, T. (1979), *Restructuring the Health Service* (London: Croom Helm).

HENCKE, D. (1985), 'Fowler advised to avoid cuts at medical schools', *The Guardian*, 1 April.

HIGGINS, J. (1983), 'Collaboration with the private sector: problems from district health authorities', *Public Administration*, vol. 61, no.2, pp.216–20.

HIGGINS, J. (1988), *The Business of Medicine: Private Health Care in Britain* (London: Macmillan).

HIRSCHMAN, A. O. (1970), *Exit, Voice, and Loyalty* (Cambridge, MA: Harvard University Press).

HOLLAND, W. W. (1983), *Evaluation of Health Care* (Oxford: Oxford University Press).

HOOVER, K. and PLANT, R. (1989), *Conservative Capitalism in Britain and the United States* (London: Routledge).

HUNTER, D. J. (1980), *Coping with Uncertainty* (Letchworth: Research Studies Press).

HUNTER, D. J. (1982), 'Organising for health: the National Health Service in the United Kingdom', *Journal of Public Policy*, vol. 2, Part 3, pp.263–300.

HUNTER, D. J. (1983a), 'The privatisation of public provision', *The Lancet*, 4 June, pp.1264–8.

HUNTER, D. J. (1983b), 'Patterns of organisation for health: a systems overview of the NHS in the UK' in A. Williamson and G. Room (eds), *Health and Welfare States of Britain: An Inter-Country Comparison* (London: Heinemann).

HUNTER, D. J. (1983c), 'Centre-periphery relations in the NHS: facilitators or inhibitors of innovation?' in K. Young (ed.), *National Interests and Local Government*, Joint Studies in Public Policy no.7 (London: Heinemann).

HUNTER, D. J. (1984), 'The lure of the organisational fix: re-organising the Scottish Health Service' in D. McCrone (ed.), *The Scottish Government Yearbook 1985* (Edinburgh: Unit for the Study of Government in Scotland).

HUNTER, D. J. and JUDGE, K. (1988), *Griffiths and Community Care: Meeting the Challenge*, Briefing Paper no.5 (London: King's Fund Institute).

HUNTER, D. J. and WISTOW, G. (1987), *Community Care in Britain: Variations on a Theme* (London: King's Fund Institute).

HUNTER, D. J. and WISTOW, G. (1988), 'The Scottish difference: policy and practice in community care' in D. McCrone and A. Brown (eds), *The Scottish Government Yearbook 1988* (Edinburgh: Unit for the Study of Government in Scotland).

HUNTER, D. J., JUDGE, K. and PRICE, S. (1988), *Community Care:*

Reacting to Griffiths, Briefing Paper no.1 (London: King's Fund Institute).
JACKSON, P. M. (1985), 'Perspectives on practical monetarism' in P. M. Jackson (ed.), Implementing Government Policy Initiatives: The Thatcher Administration 1979–83 (London: Royal Institute of Public Administration).
JENKINS, L., BARDSLEY, M., COLES, J., WICKINGS, I., and LEOW, H. (1987), Use and Validity of NHS Performance Indicators – A National Survey (London: CASPE Research/King's Fund Institute).
JOINT WORKING PARTY (1967) (Chairman: Mr. G. P. E. Howard), The Shape of Hospital Management in 1980? (London: King Edward's Hospital Fund for London).
JONES, P. R. (1981), Doctors in the BMA: A Case Study in Collective Action (Farnborough: Gower).
JUDGE, K. (1982), 'The growth and decline of social expenditure' in A. Walker (ed.) Public Expenditure and Social Policy (London: Heinemann).
KEYNES, J. M. (1936), The General Theory of Employment, Interest and Money (London: Macmillan).
KING'S FUND (1988), The Nation's Health (London: King Edward's Hospital Fund for London).
KING'S FUND INSTITUTE (1987), Public Expenditure and the NHS: Trends and Prospects (London: King Edward's Hospital Fund for London).
KING'S FUND INSTITUTE (1988), Health Finance: Assessing the Options, Briefing Paper no.4 (London: King Edward's Hospital Fund for London).
KING'S FUND INSTITUTE (1989), Efficiency in the NHS: A Study of Cost Improvement Programmes, (A joint study by a working group from the King's Fund Institute, IHSM, and NAHA) (London: King Edward's Hospital Fund for London).
KING'S FUND WORKING PARTY (1977), (Chairman: Dr. Bryan Thwaites), The Education and Training of Senior Managers in the National Health Service (London: King Edward's Hospital Fund for London).
KLEIN, R. E. (1974a), 'Policy making in the National Health Service', Political Studies, vol. 22, no.1, pp.1–14.
KLEIN, R. E. (1974b), 'Policy problems and policy perceptions in the National Health Service', Policy and Politics, vol. 2, no.3, pp.219–36.
KLEIN, R. E. (1981), 'Health services' in P. M. Jackson (ed.), Government Policy Initiatives 1979–80 (London: Royal Institute of Public Administration).
KLEIN, R. E. (1982a), 'Private practice and public policy: regulating the frontiers' in G. McLachlan and A. Maynard (eds), The Public/Private Mix for Health (London: Nuffield Provincial Hospitals Trust).
KLEIN, R. E. (1982b), 'Performance evaluation and the NHS: a case study in conceptual perplexity and organisational complexity', Public Administration, vol. 60, no.4, pp.385–407.
KLEIN, R. E. (1983), The Politics of the National Health Service (London: Longman).
KLEIN, R. E. (1984), 'The politics of ideology vs. the reality of politics:

the case of Britain's National Health Service in the 1980s', *Millbank Memorial Fund Quarterly: Health and Society*, vol. 62, no.1, pp.82–109.

KLEIN, R. E. (1985), 'Health policy 1979–83: the retreat from ideology?' in P. M. Jackson (ed.), *Implementing Government Policy Initiatives: The Thatcher Administration 1979–83* (London: Royal Institute of Public Administration).

KLEIN, R. E and LEWIS, J. (1976), *The Politics of Consumer Representation* (London: Centre for Studies in Social Policy).

KOGAN, M., GOODWIN, B., HENKEL, M., KORMAN, M., PACKWOOD, T., BUSH, A., HOYES, V., ASH, L. and TESTER, J. (1978), *The Working of the National Health Service*, Royal Commission of the National Health Service, Research Paper no.1. (London: HMSO).

LAING, W. (1988), *Review of Private Healthcare 1988* (London: Laing and Buisson).

LAND, T. (1987), 'Doctors on the Scrap Heap', *Health Service Journal*, vol. 97, no.5062, p.97.

LARKIN, G. V. (1983), *Occupational Monopoly and Modern Medicine* (London: Tavistock).

LEE, K. (1982), 'Public Expenditure, Health Services and Health' in A. Walker (ed.), *Public Expenditure and Social Policy* (London: Heinemann).

LEE, K. and MILLS, A. (1982), *Policy-Making and Planning in the Health Sector* (London: Croom Helm).

LEVITT, R. and WALL, A. (1984), *The Reorganized National Health Service* (London: Croom Helm).

LINDBLOM, C. E. (1959), 'The science of muddling through', *Public Administration Review*, vol. 19, no.3, pp.79–88.

LINDBLOM, C. E. (1977), *Politics and Markets* (New York: Basic Books).

LINDBLOM, C. E. (1979), 'Still muddling, not yet through', *Public Administration Review*, vol. 39, no.6, pp.517–26.

LIPSKY, M. (1980), *Street-Level Bureaucracy* (New York: Russell Sage Foundation).

LONG, A. F., MERCER, G., BROOKS, F., HARRISON, S., RATHWELL, T. and BARNARD, K. (1987), *Health Manpower: Planning, Production and Management* (London: Croom Helm).

LOWE, H. (1988), 'The Health Service: problems and policies', *Interlink*, Special Issue no.8, p.34.

LUKES, S. (1977), *Essays in Social Theory* (London: Macmillan).

MARCH, J.G. (1978), 'Bounded rationality, ambiguity, and the engineering of human choice', *Bell Journal of Economics*, vol. 9, pp.587–608.

MARKS, L. (1988), *Promoting Better Health? An Analysis of the Government's Programme for Improving Primary Care*, Briefing Paper no.7 (London: King's Fund Institute).

MARTIN, F. M. (1984), *Between the Acts: Community Mental Health Services 1959–1983* (London: Nuffield Provincial Hospitals Trust).

MAXWELL, R. (1981), *Health and Wealth: An International Study of Health Care Spending* (Lexington: MA, Lexington Books).

MAYNARD, A. (1983), 'Privatising the National Health Service' *Lloyds Bank Review*, no.148, pp.28–41.
MAYNARD, A. (1984), 'Private practice: answer or irrelevance?', *British Medical Journal*, vol. 288, pp.1849–51.
MAYNARD, A. (1986), 'The National Health Service: An Annual Report' in D. Mayston and F. Terry (eds), *Public Domain* (London: Public Finance Foundation).
MAYS, N. (1987), 'Measuring need in the National Health Service resource allocation formula: standardised mortality ratios or social deprivation?' *Public Administration*, vol. 65, no.1, pp.45–60.
McINNES, D. (1987), 'Medical and dental staffing prospects in the NHS in England and Wales in 1986', *Health Trends*, vol. 19, no.3, pp.1–8.
→ McKEOWN, T. (1980), *The Role of Medicine: Dream, Mirage or Nemesis?* (2nd edition) (Oxford: Blackwell).
MICHELS, R. (1915), *Political Parties* (London: Constable).
MILLAR, B. (1988), 'Achieving a balance – counting the cost', *Health Service Journal*, 24 October, p.1383.
MILLS, I. (1987), 'Regional realism: reaping rewards', *Health Service Journal*, 23 April, pp.470–1.
MINISTRY OF HEALTH AND SCOTTISH HOME AND HEALTH DEPARTMENT (1966) (Chairman: Mr. Brian Salmon), *Report of the Committee on Senior Nursing Staff Structure* (London: HMSO).
MOORE, W. (1989), 'Snubbed GPs seek talks in wake of contract poll', *Health Service Journal*, 27 July, p.899.
MULKAY, M., ASHMORE, M. and PINCH, T. (1987), 'Measuring the quality of life: a sociological invention concerning the application of economics to health care', *Sociology*, vol. 21, no.4, pp.541–64.
NAHA (1989), *The NHS Handbook* (4th edition) (London: Macmillan).
NAIRNE, P. (1983), 'Managing the DHSS elephant: reflections on a giant department', *Political Quarterly*, vol. 54, no.3, pp.243–56.
NATIONAL AUDIT OFFICE (1986), *Report by the Comptroller and Auditor General: Value for Money Developments in the National Health Service* (London: HMSO).
NATIONAL AUDIT OFFICE (1987), *Community Care Developments* (London: HMSO).
NATIONAL AUDIT OFFICE (1988), *Quality of Clinical Care in National Health Service Hospitals*, HC 736 (London: HMSO).
NATIONAL HEALTH SERVICE MANAGEMENT INQUIRY (1983), *Report* ('The Griffiths Report') (London: Department of Health and Social Security).
NAVARRO, V. (1984), 'The crisis of the international capitalist order and its implications on the welfare state' in J. B. McKinlay (ed.), *Issues in the Political Economy of Health Care* (London: Tavistock).
NICHOLL, J. P., WILLIAMS, B. T., THOMAS, K. J. and KNOWELDEN, J. (1984), 'Contribution of the private sector to elective surgery in England and Wales', *Lancet*, no. 8394, pp.89–92.
NISKANEN, W. A. (1971), *Bureaucracy and Representative Government* (Chicago: Aldine-Atherton).
O'CONNOR, J. (1973), *The Fiscal Crisis of the State* (New York: St

Martin's Press).
OECD (1985), *Measuring Health Care 1960-83* (Paris: Organisation for Economic Co-operation and Development).
OECD (1987), *Financing and Delivering Health Care* (Paris: Organisation for Economic Co-operation and Development).
OFFE, C. (1984), *Contradictions of the Welfare State* (edited and translated by J. Keane) (London: Hutchinson).
OFFE, C. (1985), *Disorganized Capitalism* (Cambridge: Polity Press).
OFFICE OF HEALTH ECONOMICS (1987), *Compendium of Health Statistics* (6th edition) (London: Office of Health Economics).
O'HIGGINS, M. (1987), *Health Spending: A Way to Sustainable Growth* (London: Institute of Health Services Management).
OPCS (1987), *Population Trends no.47* (London: OPCS).
OPEN UNIVERSITY (1988), *D321: Professional Judgement* (Milton Keynes: Open University Press).
PATER, J. E. (1981), *The Making of the National Health Service* (London: King's Fund Institute).
PATTEN, J. and POLLITT, C. J. (1980), 'Power and rationality: theories of policy formation', Paper 8 in *D336 Policies, People and Administration* (Milton Keynes: Open University Press).
PEACH, L. (1988), 'Making changes with a dose of politics', *Health Service Journal*, 14 January, pp.42–3.
PEET, J. (1987), *Health Competition: How to Improve the NHS*, Policy Study no.86 (London: Centre for Policy Studies).
PERRIN, J. (1988), *Resource Management in the NHS* (Wokingham, Berks: Van Nostrand Reinhold).
PHILLIPSON, C. (1988), *Planning for Community Care: Facts and Fallacies in the Griffiths Report*, Working Paper no.1 (Keele, Staffs: University of Keele Centre for Social Gerontology).
PINCH, T., MULKAY, M., and ASHMORE, M. (1989), 'Clinical budgeting: experimentation in the social sciences: a drama in five acts', *Accounting Organisations and Society*, vol. 14, no.3, pp.271–301.
POLLITT, C. J. (1984a), *Manipulating the Machine: Changing the Pattern of Ministerial Departments 1960-83* (London: Allen and Unwin).
POLLITT, C. J. (1984b), 'Inequalities in health care', Unit 12 in *D355 Social Policy and Social Welfare* (Milton Keynes: Open University Press).
POLLITT, C. J. (1985a), 'Measuring performance: a new system for the National Health Service', *Policy and Politics*, vol. 13, no.1, pp.1–15.
POLLITT, C. J. (1985b), 'Can practice be made perfect?', *Health and Social Service Journal*, 6 June, pp.706–7.
POLLITT, C. J. (1986a), 'Models of policy implementation: the case of the NHS', *Teaching Politics*, vol. 15, no.3, pp.445–58.
POLLITT, C. J. (1986b), 'Beyond the managerial model: the case for broadening performance assessment in government and the public services', *Financial Accountability and Management*, vol. 2, no.3, pp.155–70.
POLLITT, C. J. (1987), 'Capturing quality? The quality issue in British and American health care policies', *Journal of Public Policy*, vol. 7, no.1, pp.71–92.

POLLITT, C. J. (1988), 'Bringing consumers into performance measurement: concepts, consequences and constraints', *Policy and Politics*, vol. 16, no.2, pp.77–87.
POLLITT, C. J. (1990), *Managerialism and the Public Services: The Anglo-American Experience* (Oxford: Blackwell).
POLLITT, C. J., HARRISON, S., HUNTER, D. J. and MARNOCH, G. (1988), 'The reluctant managers: clinicians and budgets in the NHS', *Financial Accountability and Management*, vol. 4, no.3, pp.213–233.
POULANTZAS, N. (1978), *State, Power, Socialism* (London: New Left Books).
POWELL, J. E. (1976), *Medicine and Politics: 1975 and After* (London: Pitman Medical).
RANADÉ, W. (1985), 'Motives and behaviour in district health authorities', *Public Administration*, vol. 63, no.2, pp.183–200.
RATHWELL, T. A. (1987), *Strategic Planning in the Health Sector* (London: Croom Helm).
REGIONAL CHAIRMEN (1976), *Enquiry into the Working of the DHSS in Relation to Regional Health Authorities* (London: Department of Health and Social Security).
RESEARCH UNIT IN HEALTH AND BEHAVIOURAL CHANGE (1989), *Changing the Public Health* (Chichester: Wiley and Sons).
RESOURCE ALLOCATION WORKING PARTY (1976), *Sharing Resources for Health in England* (London: HMSO).
RHODES, R. A. W. (1988), *Beyond Westminster and Whitehall: Sub-Central Government in the United Kingdom* (London: Allen and Unwin).
RIVLIN, A. (1971), *Systematic Thinking for Social Action* (Washington D.C.: Brookings Institution).
ROYAL COLLEGE OF GENERAL PRACTITIONERS (1985), *What Sort of Doctor? Assessing Quality of Care in General Practice* (London: RCPG).
ROYAL COMMISSION ON THE NATIONAL HEALTH SERVICE (1979), (Chairman: Sir Alec Merrison), *Report*, Cmnd.7615 (London: HMSO).
SCHMITTER, P. C. (1974), 'Still the century of corporatism?' *Review of Politics*, vol. 36, pp.85–131.
SCHULZ, R. I. and HARRISON, S. (1983), *Teams and Top Managers in the NHS: a Survey and a Strategy*, Project Paper no. 41 (London: King's Fund).
SCOTTISH HEALTH MANAGEMENT EFFICIENCY GROUP (1987), *Income Generation: Action Plan 4* (Edinburgh: SHMEG).
SCOTTISH HEALTH SERVICES COUNCIL (1966) (Chairman: Mr. W. M. Farquharson-Lang), *Administrative Practice of Hospital Boards in Scotland* (Edinburgh: HMSO).
SCOTTISH HOME AND HEALTH DEPARTMENT (1976), *The Way Ahead* (Edinburgh: HMSO).
SCOTTISH HOME AND HEALTH DEPARTMENT (1980), *Scottish Health Authorities Priorities for the Eighties* (Edinburgh: HMSO).
SCOTTISH HOME AND HEALTH DEPARTMENT (1988), *Scottish Health Authorities Revised Priorities for the Eighties and Nineties* (Edin-

burgh: HMSO).
SEIBERT, W. (1977), 'Occupational licensing: the Merrison Report on the regulation of the medical profession', *British Journal of Industrial Relations*, vol. XV, no.1, pp.29–38.
SELDON, A. (ed.) (1980), *The Litmus Papers: A National Health Disservice* (London: Centre for Policy Studies).
SHAW, C. D. (1986), *Quality Assurance: What the Colleges are Doing* (London: King's Fund).
SHORE, E. (1974), 'Medical Manpower Planning', *Health Trends*, vol. 6, no.2, pp.32–35.
SMITH, D. J. (1980), *Overseas Doctors in the National Health Service* (London: Policy Studies Institute).
SOCIAL SERVICES COMMITTEE (1981), *Fourth Report, Session 1980-81: Medical Manpower with Special Reference to the Number of Doctors and the Career Structure in Hospitals* (London: House of Commons/HMSO).
SOCIAL SERVICES COMMITTEE (1984), *First Report, Session 1983-84: Griffiths NHS Management Inquiry Report*, HC 209 (London: House of Commons/HMSO).
SOCIAL SERVICES COMMITTEE (1985), *Fifth Report, Session 1984-85: Medical Education Report: Follow-Up* (London: House of Commons/HMSO).
SOCIAL SERVICES COMMITTEE (1986), *Fourth Report, Session 1985-86: Public Expenditure on the Social Services* (in two volumes) (London: House of Commons/HMSO).
SOCIAL SERVICES COMMITTEE (1988), *Sixth Report, Session 1987-88: Public Expenditure on the Social Services* (London: HMSO).
SOCIAL SERVICES COMMITTEE (1989), *Eighth Report, Session 1988-89: Resourcing the National Health Service: the Government's Plans for the future of the National Health Service*, HC 214-III (London: HMSO).
STANDING COMMISSION ON PAY COMPARABILITY (1979) (Chairman: Prof. H. A. Clegg), *Report No.1: Local Authority and University Manual Workers; NHS Ancillary Staffs; and Ambulancemen*, Cmnd.7641 (London: HMSO).
STANDING COMMISSION ON PAY COMPARABILITY (1980) (Chairman: Prof. H. A. Clegg), *Report No.4: Professions Supplementary to Medicine*, Cmnd.7850 (London: HMSO).
STEERING GROUP FOR IMPLEMENTATION (1987), *Hospital Medical Staffing – Achieving a Balance: A Plan for Action* (London: UK Health Departments).
STEVENS, R. (1966), *Medical Practice in Modern England: The Impact of Specialisation and State Medicine* (New Haven, CT: Yale University Press).
STEWART, R., SMITH, P., BLAKE, J. and WINGATE, P. (1980), *The District Administration in the National Health Service* (London: King's Fund Institute).
STOCKING, B. (1985), *Initiative and Inertia: Case Studies in the NHS* (London: Nuffield Provincial Hospitals Trust).
STOWE, K. (1989), *On Caring for the National Health: The Rock Carling Fellowship 1988* (London: Nuffield Provincial Hospitals Trust).

TAYLOR-GOOBY, P. (1985), 'The politics of welfare: public attitudes and behaviour' in R. E. Klein and M. O'Higgins (eds), *The Future of Welfare* (Oxford: Blackwell).
THOMPSON, D. J. C. (1986), *Coalition and Decision-Making Within Health Districts*, Research Report no.23 (Birmingham: University of Birmingham Health Services Management Centre).
THWAITES, B. (1987), *The NHS: the End of the Rainbow* (Southampton: University of Southampton Institute of Health Policy Studies).
TIMMINS, N. (1989), 'Clarke waters down cut-throat NHS price competition', *Independent*, 28 June, p.8.
TOLLIDAY, H. (1978), 'Clinical autonomy' in E. Jacques (ed.), *Health Services: Their Nature and Organisation and the Role of Patients, Doctors, and the Health Professions* (London: Heinemann).
TOWNSEND, P. and DAVIDSON, N. (eds) (1983), *Inequalities in Health: the Black Report* (Harmondsworth: Penguin Books).
WARNER, N. (1984), 'Raynerism in practice: anatomy of a Rayner scrutiny', *Public Administration*, vol. 62, no.1, pp.7–22.
WATKIN, B. (1975), *Documents on Health and Social Services: 1834 to the Present Day* (London: Methuen).
WATKIN, B. (1978), *The National Health Service: The First Phase – 1948–1974 and After* (London: Allen and Unwin).
WEINER, S. L., MAXWELL, J. H., SAPOLSKY, H. M., DUNN, D. L. and HSIAO, W. C. (1987), 'Economic incentives and organisational realities: managing hospitals under DRGs', *Milbank Quarterly*, vol. 65, no.4, pp.463–487.
WELSH OFFICE (1976), *Proposed All-Wales Policies and Priorities for the Planning and Provision of Health and Personal Social Services from 1976/77 to 1979/80: A Consultative Document* (Cardiff: HMSO).
WELSH OFFICE (1980), *The Structure and Management of the NHS in Wales* (Cardiff: HMSO).
WHITEHEAD, M. (1987), *The Health Divide: Inequalities in Health in the 1980s* (London: Health Education Council).
WILLCOCKS, A. J. (1967), *The Creation of the National Health Service* (London: Routledge and Kegan Paul).
WILLIAMS, B. (1987), Personal communication to D. J. Hunter.
WISEMAN, C. (1979) 'Strategic planning in the Scottish Health Service – a mixed-scanning approach', *Long Range Planning*, vol. 12, pt.2, pp.103–13.
WISTOW, G. (1985), 'Community care for the mentally handicapped: disappointing progress' in A. Harrison and J. Gretton (eds), *Health Care United Kingdom 1985* (London: CIPFA).
WOOD, N. (1982), 'BMA split in major row over junior doctors' jobs', *Times Health Supplement*, 15 January, p.2.
WORKING GROUP ON JOINT PLANNING (1985), *Progress in Partnership* (London: Department of Health and Social Security).
WORLD HEALTH ORGANIZATION (1985), *Targets for Health for All* (Copenhagen: WHO Regional Office for Europe).

WRIGHT, M. (1988), 'Policy community, policy network, and comparative industrial policies', *Political Studies*, vol. 36, no.4, pp.593–612.
ZIGLIO, E. (1986), 'Uncertainty and innovation in health promotion; nutrition policy in two countries', *Health Promotion*, vol 1, pp.257–269.

Index

accountability issues 80, 86, 129
administrative and clerical staff 93
   pay 98
administrative costs, in public and private sectors 146
AIDS 67
   joint finance initiatives 35
   treatments debate 141
ambulance service 96–7, 132
   pay 99
ancillary workers 96, 97
   pay 98, 101
   pay review arrangements 99
annual independent reviews 95
arbitration, in pay disputes 95
Association of Community Health Councils 16
attitudes, to NHS 8, 39, 137–8
Audit Commission, report on community care 63
Australia 42

bargaining, in policy formation 5, 114, 149, 155
Bevan, A. 72
breast screening services 67
British Medical Association 16, 80, 85, 96, 110, 114
budgeting, by doctors 82, 171
BUPA 16
bureaucracy
   of public sector 19, 20, 21
   of state intervention 15, 19

capitalist system, provision of public health care 150, 159
career structure
   managerial 76
   medical 105–9
central government
   centre–periphery relations 86, 89, 113
   control and management reforms 91–2
   efficiency and cost-effectiveness priorities 121, 144, 146
   funding and control 87
   relationship with medical profession 148–9
   see also Cabinet; Conservative government; Labour government
Central Manpower Committee 110
cervical screening services 67
charges 45, 70, 164
charitable institutions, health care services 52
Chartered Society of Physiotherapy 96
chief executive post proposals 77, 78
chief officers 83
choice, of the individual 18, 20, 48
circulars
   ineffectiveness 1
   resources, priorities and planning 67–8
Clegg Commission 99
closed shop agreements 96
collaboration
   between health and local authorities 62
   between private and public sectors 54, 55
collective bargaining 94
commercial activities, in hospitals 47
community care 3, 61–2, 88
   failure of 62–3
   Griffiths report recommendations 63–4, 172–4
   in Scotland 65
   in Wales 65–6, 132
   joint finance initiatives 35
   role of social service departments 69, 173–4
Community Health Councils 103, 165, 176
community health services, cash-limited funds 34
community physicians 107
competition 20
   between hospital services 75, 145
   between elites 24–5
   effects on standards 145–6
   in public choice theory 90
   tendering 20, 47–8, 86, 99, 149

complaints 103, 135
computer data 143
  impact on evaluation process 151
Confederation of British Industry 80, 155
Confidential Enquiry into Perioperative Deaths 132-3
consensus management teams 77, 79
  criticisms 78, 80
Conservative government
  consultative document 1979 79
  modern management ethos 75
  NHS Management Executive 82
  NHS Policy Board 82
  public expenditure controls 33, 38
  views on NHS management 83-4, 101-2, 156, 162
  see also Thatcher administration
consultants
  health authorities views of 112, 113
  in medical career structure 105-9
  influence 12, 115, 157
  ratio to junior doctors 107, 109-12
  salaries 99
  status 107
  sub-consultant grade 109
consumers
  choice 20-1, 48
  expectation 41, 43
  health care records 144
  ineffectiveness 147, 152
  influence 119, 125
  of private sector services 53
  priority groups 61, 67
  public popularity of NHS 8, 39
  surveys 137-8
  see also patients
consumer organisations 7, 148, 176
  initiatives 149
contracting out
  of deputising services 146
  of hospital services 20, 47-8, 99
  of treatment services 172
corporate power 15, 16, 17
corporate rationalization 158
corporatism 23
  'ideological' 24
cost-effectiveness 119, 120
  as government priority 121
cost improvement programmes 37, 46, 56, 86, 149
costs
  in health care policies 71, 85-6, 126
  of administration 146
  of NHS workforce 93

of monitoring and evaluation 143
cure, concept of 118, 141

decentralization, of NHS responsibilities 85, 86
decision-making
  incrementalist 8-9, 10, 103-4
  in health authorities 77
  rational-comprehensive model 8, 10
defence 39
demand, for health care services 32-3, 41, 43
democratic process 15, 'direct' 29
demographic structure
  impact of changes 2, 35-6, 39
  resource allocation variations 72-3
  trends calculation methodology 36
Denmark 42
dental treatment 70
Department of Health 16, 165
  community care plans 64
  efficiency strategies 37
  health expenditure plans 34
  health services supervisory board 166
  income generation unit 47
  NHS management board 166, 169
  NHS policy board 169
Department of Health & Social Security 165
  circular on resources, priorities amd planning 67-8
  control over NHS 83
  effectiveness of circulars 1
  efficiency monitoring 147-8
  medical staffing discussions 111
  ministerial reviews of RHAs 128-9
  relationship with commercial companies 16, 147
  relationships with health authorities 81, 146
dependency 1
  networks 2
depoliticizing, of NHS management 85
deputizing services, commercial 146
direct democracy 29
district health authorities 20, 167
  review process 128
  role 170, 176
doctor-patient relationship 145
doctors
  as a 'professional monopoly' 25, 91, 102, 116, 158
  'clinical freedom' 102-3, 115
  emigration opportunity decline 107
  immigrant 108, 109

pay 98–9, 101, 102
  role in management budgeting 82
  training 105–6
  workload related budgets 168
  see also consultants; hospital doctors
drug abuse 2
  misusers services 67
drugs, cost control 16

economic factors
  in health care financing 2, 38, 42, 163
  in modification of elitist structures 161
economic policies 37–8
Economic & Social Research Council 136, 145
education 19, 42
  vouchers 48
  see also medical education
effectiveness
  of NHS 118, 121, 144
  of preventive services 71, 144
efficiency 119
  and ownership status 145
  DoH programmes 37, 86, 149
  incentives 90
  in resource allocation 41–2, 75, 85–6
  measurement 126
  savings 80
  through management controls 84–5
elderly
  community care needs 64
  effects of increasing population 2, 35–6, 43, 73
  GP regular care service 71
  private residential care 51
elite theory 22, 24–6, 159
  see also neo-elitism
elites
  economic influences on structure 161
  emerging managerial 91, 158, 161
  power 22–3, 58
Elizabeth Garrett Anderson Hospital 98
Ely geriatric hospital 124
emigration 109
  opportunities decline 107
employment incentives, private health care insurance as 50
England
  health care expenditure 40
  NHS organization 2
environment issues 42
evaluation
  as political issue 151–2
  criteria 118–20

  key developments in 128
  methods 127–38
  of NHS services 123–7
  political theory perspectives 120–3, 145–50
  problems 138–44
eye tests 70

family, caring roles 62, 64
Family Practitioner Committees 135, 165, 168, 170–1
family practitioner services 71, 130
  open-ended funds 34
Farquharson-Lang Report on Scottish hospital administration 76, 77
finance of NHS 33–5, 37, 39, 44, 162–3, 164, 165–6
  supplementary 45–9
  under- 41–3
foodstuffs, health effects 16, 70
Fowler, N. 80
France 42
fund-raising activities 46, 47

General Medical Council 1, 106
general practice
  compulsory vocational training scheme 106, 108
  evaluation 134–5
  'indicative' prescribing budgets 171
  practice budgets 171
general practitioners 1
  assessment 134
  incentives for preventive health care 70–1, 135, 171
  in medical career structure 105–7, 108
  new contracts 117, 135
  self-employment 102
  training 106, 108
  use of private sector 53
Godber Report 110
Greece 42
Griffiths, R. 60, 63, 80, 125
Griffiths Report on community care 63–4, 69
  government response to 64, 69
Griffiths Report on NHS management 8, 60, 78, 80, 83, 103, 104, 125, 166
  conclusions and recommendations 81, 82, 84, 166
gross domestic product (GDP), and health care expenditure 34

Index 197

Guillebaud Committee on NHS
 expenditure 126

Halsbury Committees 98
health
 definitions 138, 139–40
 individualistic perspective 70
 medical model of 8, 140
 social deprivation factors 41, 73–4
Health & Medicines Act 1988 47, 54
health administrators 76
Health Advisory Service 124–5
health authorities 165
 attitude to consultant posts 112, 113, 115
 consensus management groups 77
 coordination problems with social service departments 3
 funds allocation 34–5
 impact of government circulars 1, 67–8
 increased control and responsibilities 79
 relationship with DHSS 146
 use of private sector services 54
health authority members 13
 lay 7, 77–8
 professional officers 77–8
health care managers 83, 167
 as agents of government 84
 as emerging elite 91, 158, 161
 in competitive health system 116
 individual performance reviews 135–6, 167
 role in policymaking process 7, 12, 103–4
 training 76
health care policies
 community 62–4
 determining factors 71–2
 development and implementation process 3–5, 15–16, 162–3
 local versus national 13, 157
 political theory perspectives 153, 154–61
 'shared version' 6–8, 31, 153
health care services 19, 172
 as basic human right 45
 centre - periphery relations 86, 89, 113
 data collection systems 143–4
 demand 35–7, 41, 43
 development 37
 devolution 86–7
 equity 119–20, 125–6
 expectations of 41, 43
 expenditure 34, 38, 40, 42, 44
 expenditure variations 40–1
 finance 32, 55–9
 geographical variations 72, 174–6
 inflation 39
 internal market concept 75, 169, 171–2
 international expenditure comparisons 42
 mixed-economy 55, 58, 65, 90, 91
 planning 61, 67–8, 175
 quality 118–19
 resources supply 37–41
 two-tier 54, 91
 see also National Health Service; private health care sector
health departments 165
 administrative differences 174–6
 controls over resources 7
 criticisms 81
health education programmes 143
health insurance schemes 49
health promotion, as policy 69, 70, 71, 88–9
health records 143–4
Hospital Advisory Service 124
Hospital Consultants and Specialists Association 112
hospital doctors
 associate specialists 105
 consultant:junior ratios 107–12
 hospital practitioner grade 112
 junior 105, 112, 117
hospital record systems 123
hospitals
 cash-limited funds 34
 closure 97–8
 district 167
 Griffiths recommendations 170
 hospital revenue allocation formula 73
 impact of competition 105
 income-generating schemes 47, 132
 planning 61
 regional provision variations 72
 self-governing proposals 20, 104, 170
 see also private hospitals
housing 41
hypothecation 45–6

ideological corporatism 24, 115, 116, 158
immigrant junior hospital doctors 108, 109
incentives

for GPs 135, 171
in internal market concept 75
income-generating schemes 46–7
incremental analysis 9, 12, 103–4, 154
incremental politics 9, 11, 12, 91, 103, 157
incrementalism 6, 8–9, 114
degrees of 11
limitations of 12–13
Individual Performance Reviews 135–6
industrial disputes 96–7
outcome 97–101
industrial relations 94–101
effects of White Paper 104–5
inequality
and role of the state 27–8
in distribution of resources 73
inflation
impact on public spending 38–9
in health services 39
informal care 62, 64
information
for health services consumers 53, 135
health-relevant 144
systems 143
inner city areas, over-provision 73
inspectorate 124–5
Institute of Health Services Management 44
Institute of Hospital Administrators 76
interdependency 1
of private and public health care sectors 53–4
internal market concept 20, 54, 75, 169, 171–2
Italy 42

Japan 42
Jenkin, P. 115
Joint Consultants Committee 110
joint financing 35
joint planning, for community care 62–3
Joint Planning Advisory Committee 111

King's Fund 77
Korner reports 143

Labour government, expenditure controls 37–8
laissez-faire philosophy 86
lay persons, weak position of 7
liberal corporatism 23, 114, 115, 122, 157

management budgeting 82, 168
management of the NHS 75–87, 165
central control strategies 129
consensus management concept 77, 78–9
efficiency strategies 60, 83, 166
Griffiths Report recommendations 60, 81–2, 84, 169
political perspectives 88–92
priority setting 61–72
problems 61, 87
reorganization 78–9, 165
see also health care managers
management theory 88
managerial relations 93, 101–4, 113
manual workers 93
market relations 93
impact of changes in workforce relations 97–101
Marxism 26, 30, 150
see also neo-Marxism
medical advances
impact on objectives and priorities 67, 139
impact on resource allocation 36
medical assistant 109, 110
medical audit committees 133, 148
medical care, evaluation problems 124, 141
medical education 106, 144–5
funding 117
medical manpower issues 107, 109–12
political theory perspectives 113–16
politics of 112–13
see also career structure
medical profession
as an elite 23–4, 26, 57–8, 115, 148, 159
autonomy 91
Central Manpower Committee 110
defensive stance 7, 115
divisions within 26
health definition 140
influences 102, 113–17
managerial influences 103–4
monitoring initiatives 132–5
pay 98
relationship with government 115, 148–9
relationship with public 58
Medical Research Council, Epidemiology Unit 124
Medicare 22
mentally handicapped, All Wales Strategy for the Development of

Index

Services for Mentally Handicapped People 65–6
mentally ill, community care in Scotland 65
Ministry of Health 110, 165
  see also Department of Health; Department of Health & Social Security
mixed-economy strategies, in health services 55, 58, 65, 90, 91
monitoring strategies 20, 123–4 127–38
monopoly power, of public service professions 20
moral values 18
mortality rates, perioperative 132–3

Nairn, P. 83
National Audit Office 46, 111, 123–4
National Health Service 1, 164
  administrative practices 76–7
  aims 68–9
  basic principles of 45, 50
  chief executive 82
  consultative documents 79
  'crisis' 150, 159–60
  funding 32–5, 44–5, 87, 164–5
  funding policies 56–9, 162–3
  funding requirements 37
  industrial relations 94–101
  Management Executive 82, 129, 169
  managerial relations 101–4
  Marxist view of 150, 159
  objectives 66
  occupational complexity constraints 8
  organisational structure 31, 165, 166–8
  Policy Board 82, 129, 169
  policy differences in UK 3, 174–6
  political consensus 8, 28
  priority groups 67
  public opinion 8, 39, 137–8
  reforms 84
  regional variations 151
  relationship with independent sector 53–4
  reorganization 1974 60, 78, 165
  reorganization 1982 79
  responsiveness to needs 119, 125
  supplementary finance 45–9
  under-funding 41–4
  unionisation 95–6
  workforce 93–4
  see also finance of NHS; management of NHS

National Health Service Management Inquiry 60, 166
national income, and health care spending 44
national insurance, contribution to NHS funding 33, 45–6
National Union of Public Employees 96, 101
needs 119, 125
  and resource allocation 41, 44
neo-conservatives 18
neo-elitism 22–6, 55, 56–8, 88, 89, 91, 115, 117, 122, 148–9, 157–9, 160–1
neo-liberals 18
neo-Marxism 27–30, 55, 57, 89, 91, 122–3, 149–50, 159–61
neo-pluralism 14–17, 55, 56, 88, 89, 90, 121, 147, 154–5
Netherlands 42
new left 27, 28
New Rationalism 75
new right 18, 87, 156
  and concept of internal market 20
Northern Ireland 34
  health care expenditure 40
  NHS organization 3, 79, 174–5
  NHS revenue finance 2
Norway, national nutrition and food policy 70
nuclear reprocessing plants, cancer links 143
nurses 76
  industrial disputes 97
  pay 98, 102
  shortage 2
  status 77, 148

objectives
  in policy evaluation 141
  in review process 127–8
  of individual managers 135–6
  of NHS 66, 147, 166
oligarchy, iron law of 22
organizational structure, of NHS 31, 165, 166–8, 173
  Griffiths recommendations 169–70
Owen, D. 81

Paige, V. 82
Parliament, political role in NHS 45, 155
partisan mutual adjustment system (PMA) 6–7, 9, 11–12, 114, 154
patients
  charges 45

competition for 20
cross-boundary flows 167, 170
pressure groups 62, 155
pay 98–9, 100
  and productivity 95
  incentives for GPs 135
  performance related 135–6
pay disputes 95, 96–7
  independent reviews 98–9
Peach, L. 81
performance indicators 20, 80, 86, 130–1
Performance-Related Pay 135–6, 167
performance reviews 155
  of individual managers 135–6, 167
  of regions 129
personal social services 19, 61
  see also social service departments
pharmaceutical industry 16
  relationship with DHSS 147
planning, of health care services 61, 67–8, 175
  see also health care policies
Platt Report on medical education 109
pluralism 17, 18
  definition 23
  see also neo-pluralism
policy-making process 1
  as bargaining network 2, 5
  as partisan mutual adjustment 6–7, 11–12
  constraints 2
  national level 13
  scrutinies 86
  theories of 4–5
policy networks 15
  exclusive 16
political institutions, decline in influence 15
political integration 16
political parties, consensus on NHS 8, 28, 154
political theories
  relevance for specific policy issues 14, 31, 55, 88–92, 113–16, 120–3, 145–51, 154–61
  see also neo-elitism; neo-Marxism; neo-pluralism; public choice theory
Ponting, C. 132
population, in resource allocation formulae 74–5
Powell, E. 32, 34
power relationships 1
  evaluation perspectives 120–3

government/doctor 115
  in policymaking 5, 13
  political theories of 13–30
  'shared version' 6–8
prescription charges 33, 45
preventative medicine 69, 70–1
  effects of charges 70
  GP incentives 70–1
  pricing mechanisms 54
primary health care 13, 70–1
  evaluation 134–5
  Griffiths proposals 170–1
priorities 61, 67, 142
  ranking 68
priority groups 61–2, 67, 118, 141–2
  in community care strategies 64–6
  in preventive health care 71
priority setting 66–9
  as rationing 142
private health care sector 51–4, 56
  encouragement 20, 50, 90
  flexibility 55
private health insurance 20, 49–50
  failings 51
  tax relief 45, 50
private hospitals
  ownership 52
  short-term contracts with NHS hospitals 53
private practice 79, 107
productivity, and pay 95
professional bodies
  as trade unions 96
  influence of 23–4
public accountability 32
Public Accounts Committee 79, 86, 126, 128, 165
public choice theory 17–22, 55, 56, 89, 90, 121–2, 145–7, 156–7
public expenditure 33
  controls 33, 37–8, 57
  neo-Marxist categories of 28
  prioritising 42
public expenditure plans 33–4
Public Expenditure Survey 33
Public Expenditure Survey Committee 33
public health specialists 107
public opinion
  of NHS 8, 39, 137–8, 142
  of White Paper on NHS 162
public sector
  bureaucracy 19, 146
  management 76, 87
Public Sector Borrowing Requirement 38

quality, of NHS care 118–19
radical right *see* new right
rational theory 88
Rayner, D. 131
Rayner scrutinies 80, 131–2
Reagan administration 20
regional health authorities 20, 167
  in review process 127, 128
  population and health care funding 74–5
  relationship with DHSS 81
  resource allocation formula 73
  role 169
  Thames 74
regional review system 86
registrars *see* hospital doctors
renal services 67
residential care homes 64
  private sector 52, 174
resource allocation formulae 13, 34, 41, 166
  criteria 73
  criticisms 74
Resource Allocation Working Party 13, 73, 154
resource management 82, 168, 176
resources
  allocation decision-making 44, 90, 98
  allocation variations 40–1
  community care needs 64
  demand 32
  diversion for monitoring programmes 143
  efficient use 85–6
  human 93–4
  influence of health departments 7
resources distribution 72–5
revenue cash limits 35
Review Body on Doctors' and Dentists' Remuneration 95
Review Body on nurses pay 102
review process 127–9
Royal College of General Practitioners 134
Royal College of Nursing 80, 96, 148
Royal Commission on Medical Education 109
Royal Commission on the NHS 41, 49, 51, 60, 66, 79, 111, 124

Salmon Report on nursing 76
school medical service 105, 106, 107
Scotland 34
  community care organization 65

evaluation and review procedures 151, 176
health care expenditure 40
hospital board administration 76
local health councils 176
NHS organization 2, 79, 175–6
NHS revenue finance 2, 151, 175
Scottish Health Authorities Priorities for the Eighties(SHAPE) 65
Scottish Health Authorities Review of Priorities for the Eighties and Nineties (SHARPEN) 65, 68
Scottish Health Service Management Efficiency Group 47
secretaries of state 165, 174
  health service funds allocation responsibilities 34
Secretary of State for Health 44
Secretary of State for Social Services 102
'self-government' concept 20, 104, 176
social care 69, 172
  NHS budget 173
social deprivation 73–4
social groups, equity in NHS 119–20, 125–6
social insurance 49
social security 39, 173, 174
  funding of private residential care 52, 63
social service departments 165
  community care responsibilities 65, 69, 173–4
  coordination problems with health authorities 3
Social Services Committee 39, 40, 68, 79, 86, 87, 111, 165
Social Services Inspectorate 64
social workers 65
Spain 42
spectacles, NHS voucher scheme 48
state
  as referee in group bargaining 14, 114, 149, 155
  -civil society relationship 18–19, 26–7
  intervention 15
status
  in management groups 77
  of consultants 107
Stowe, K. 44–5, 80, 82
structural interest theory 24
Sweden 42

taxation
  as major source of NHS funding 33,

44, 53, 164
hypothecated 46
incentives for private health care 20, 50
Thatcher, M. 131
views on health care 26, 28, 33, 150
Thatcher administration 20
economic strategy 57
see also White Paper on NHS
theory evaluation 4–5
timescale problems, in data evaluation 143
tobacco industry 16
Todd Report on medical education 109–10
trade unions 79, 155
consultants' 112
effects of competitive tendering 99–101
inter-union cooperation 97
membership 95
outcome of activities 97–9, 101
Trades Union Congress 97
training posts
in medical career structure 105–6
transport services 42
Treasury 79
concerns over NHS budget 83–4, 86
public expenditure planning 33–4
treatment contracts 172
treatment costs
and expenditure requirements 36

United Kingdom
health care funding theory 55–9
health policy variations 2–3, 88, 89, 174–6
health services expenditure 40, 42–3, 58
public spending and GDP 33, 43
see also England; Northern Ireland; Scotland; Wales
United States of America
health expenditure as % GDP 42
medical corporations 56
Medicare prospective payment system failure 22
moral majority movement 18
public finance of health care 51

see also Reagan administration 20

values
in prioritizing 139, 141
in public choice theory 18
influence in policy-making 3
vocational training scheme, for general practitioners 106, 108
voucher schemes 48

wages and salaries 35
see also pay
waiting lists 35
as evaluative indicator 140–1
reduction strategies 53, 140
Wales 2, 34, 68
community care policies 65–6, 132
consultant contracts 151
consultative document 79
health care expenditure 40
Health Planning Forum 175
Health Policy Board 175
welfare state
negative effects of 20
neo-liberal hostility 18, 19
see also National Health Service
West Germany 42
White Paper on community care 64, 172–4
White Paper on preventative health care 70, 71, 134–5
White Paper on NHS 1989 9, 20, 40, 41, 53, 56, 60–1, 71, 86, 149
impact on industrial relations 104–5
impact on medical influence 116–17
implementation issues 162, 176
opposition to 84
proposals 169–72
Whitley Councils 94–5, 98, 102, 170
women
cancer screening services 67
workforce of NHS 93–4, 155
pay 98–9, 100
see also medical manpower issues
Working for Patients see White Paper on NHS
World Health Organization
health definition 139
Health for All initiative 69, 71, 89